Asthma: Screening, Diagnosis, and Management

Editor

KAREN H. CALHOUN

OTOLARYNGOLOGIC CLINICS OF NORTH AMERICA

www.oto.theclinics.com

February 2014 • Volume 47 • Number 1

ELSEVIER

1600 John F. Kennedy Boulevard • Suite 1800 • Philadelphia, Pennsylvania, 19103-2899

http://www.oto.theclinics.com

OTOLARYNGOLOGIC CLINICS OF NORTH AMERICA Volume 47, Number 1
February 2014 ISSN 0030-6665, ISBN-13: 978-0-323-26674-1

Editor: Joanne Husovski
Development Editor: Susan Showalter

Otolaryngologic Clinics of North America (ISSN 0030-6665) is published bimonthly by Elsevier, Inc., 360 Park Avenue South, New York, NY 10010-1710. Months of issue are February, April, June, August, October, and December. Business and Editorial Offices: 1600 John F. Kennedy Blvd., Suite 1800, Philadelphia, PA 19103-2899. Customer Service Office: 6277 Sea Harbor Drive, Orlando, FL 32887-4800. Periodicals postage paid at New York, NY and additional mailing offices. Subscription prices is $365.00 per year (US individuals), $692.00 per year (US institutions), $175.00 per year (US student/resident), $485.00 per year (Canadian individuals), $876.00 per year (Canadian institutions), $540.00 per year (international individuals), $876.00 per year (international institutions), $270.00 per year (international & Canadian student/resident). Foreign air speed delivery is included in all *Clinics*' subscription prices. All prices are subject to change without notice. **POSTMASTER:** Send address changes to *Otolaryngologic Clinics of North America*, Elsevier Health Sciences Division, Subscription Customer Service, 3251 Riverport Lane, Maryland Heights, MO 63043. **Telephone: 1-800-654-2452 (U.S. and Canada); 314-447-8871 (outside U.S. and Canada). Fax: 314-447-8029. E-mail: journalscustomerservice-usa@elsevier.com (for print support); journalsonlinesupport-usa@elsevier.com (for online support).**

Reprints. For copies of 100 or more of articles in this publication, please contact the Commercial Reprints Department, Elsevier Inc., 360 Park Avenue South, New York, NY 10010-1710. Tel.: 212-633-3874; Fax: 212-633-3820; E-mail: reprints@elsevier.com.

Otolaryngologic Clinics of North America is also published in Spanish by McGraw-Hill Interamericana Editores S.A., P.O. Box 5-237, 06500 Mexico D.F., Mexico.

Otolaryngologic Clinics of North America is covered in *MEDLINE/PubMed (Index Medicus), Current Contents/Clinical Medicine, Excerpta Medica, BIOSIS, Science Citation Index,* and *ISI/BIOMED.*

Printed and bound by CPI Group (UK) Ltd, Croydon, CR0 4YY

Transferred to digital print 2013

Contributors

EDITOR

KAREN H. CALHOUN, MD, FACS, FAAOA
Professor, Department of Otolaryngology - Head and Neck Surgery, Wexner Medical Center, The Ohio State University College of Medicine, Columbus, Ohio

AUTHORS

PATRICK R. AGUILAR, MD
Department of Internal Medicine, Washington University, St Louis, Missouri

CATHY BENNINGER, RN, MS, CNP
Department of Medicine, The Ohio State University Wexner Medical Center, Columbus, Ohio

ELIZABETH BOISE, RNC, BSN, AE-C
Allergy Nurse and Certified Asthma Educator, Division of Sinus and Allergy, OSU Department of Otolaryngology - Head and Neck Surgery, Wexner Medical Center at The Ohio State University, Columbus, Ohio

KAREN H. CALHOUN, MD, FACS, FAAOA
Professor, Department of Otolaryngology - Head and Neck Surgery, Wexner Medical Center, The Ohio State University College of Medicine, Columbus, Ohio

JACQUELYNNE COREY, MD
Section of Otolaryngology - Head and Neck Surgery, Department of Surgery, University of Chicago, Chicago, Illinois

BERRYLIN J. FERGUSON, MD
Professor of Otolaryngology, UPMC Mercy, University of Pittsburgh School of Medicine, Pittsburgh, Pennsylvania

JOHN A. FORNADLEY, MD, FACS, FAAOA
Clinical Associate Professor of Surgery, Penn State University, Hershey, Pennsylvania

RACHEL GEORGOPOULOS, MD
Resident, Department of Otolaryngology, Temple University Health System, Philadelphia, Pennsylvania

BRUCE R. GORDON, MA, MD, FACS, FAAOA
Otolaryngology Chairman, Cape Cod Hospital, Hyannis; Clinical Instructor, Laryngology and Otology, Harvard University, Cambridge; Senior Teaching Faculty, Massachusetts Eye and Ear Infirmary, Boston, Massachusetts

HELENE J. KROUSE, PhD, APN-BC, CORLN, FAAN
Professor of Nursing, College of Nursing, Wayne State University, Detroit, Michigan

JOHN H. KROUSE, MD, PhD
Professor and Chairman, Department of Otolaryngology - Head and Neck Surgery, Associate Dean, Graduate Medical Education, Temple University School of Medicine, Philadelphia, Pennsylvania

JESSICA KYNYK, MD
Department of Medicine, The Ohio State University Wexner Medical Center, Columbus, Ohio

JONATHAN MASLAN, MD
Department of Otolaryngology, Wake Forest School of Medicine, Winston-Salem, North Carolina

LAURA MATRKA, MD
Assistant Professor, Department of Otolaryngology - Head and Neck Surgery, The Ohio State University Wexner Medical Center, Eye and Ear Institute, Columbus; JamesCare Voice and Swallowing Disorders Clinic, Stoneridge Medical Center, Dublin, Ohio

JUSTIN C. MCCARTY, BA
Lake Erie of Osteopathic Medicine, Bradenton, Florida

JAMES W. MIMS, MD
Department of Otolaryngology, Wake Forest School of Medicine, Winston-Salem, North Carolina

LAUREN L. MURRILL, MD
Department of Otolaryngology - Head and Neck Surgery, Loyola University Medical Center, Maywood, Illinois

MICHAEL J. PARKER, MD, FAAOA
Clinical Instructor, Department of Otolaryngology and Communication Sciences, SUNY Upstate Medical University, Syracuse, New York

JONATHAN P. PARSONS, MD, MSc, FCCP
Associate Professor of Internal Medicine; Associate Director, Ohio State University Asthma Center; Co-Director, OSU Multidisciplinary Cough Program; Division of Pulmonary, Allergy, Critical Care and Sleep Medicine, Wexner Medical Center, 201 Davis Heart and Lung Research Institute, Columbus, Ohio

MONICA OBEROI PATADIA, MD
Department of Otolaryngology - Head and Neck Surgery, Loyola University Medical Center, Maywood, Illinois

MATTHEW W. RYAN, MD
Associate Professor, Department of Otolaryngology-Head and Neck Surgery, University of Texas Southwestern Medical Center, Dallas, Texas

MINKA L. SCHOFIELD, MD
Assistant Professor, Division of Sinus and Allergy, Department of Otolaryngology - Head and Neck Surgery, The Eye and Ear Institute, Wexner Medical Center, The Ohio State University, Columbus, Ohio

ELINA TOSKALA, MD, PhD
Department of Otolaryngology, Temple University Health System, Philadelphia, Pennsylvania

EVAN S. WALGAMA, MD
Department of Otolaryngology - Head and Neck Surgery, University of Texas Southwestern Medical Center, Dallas, Texas

KAREN L. WOOD, MD
Department of Medicine, The Ohio State University Wexner Medical Center, Columbus, Ohio

Contents

Consideration of the unified airway model when managing patients with
rhinitis and or asthma allows a more comprehensive care plan and therefore improved patient outcomes. Asthma is linked to rhinitis both epidemiologically and biologically, and this association is even stronger in
individuals with atopy. Rhinitis is not only associated with but is a risk factor for the development of asthma. Management of rhinitis improves
asthma control. Early and aggressive treatment of allergic rhinitis may
prevent the development of asthma. In patients with allergic rhinitis
that is not sufficiently controlled by allergy medication, allergen-directed
immunotherapy should be considered.

Asthma is an obstructive pulmonary disorder with exacerbations characterized by symptoms of shortness of breath, cough, chest tightness,
and/or wheezing. Symptoms are caused by chronic airway inflammation.
There are multiple cell types and inflammatory mediators involved in its
pathophysiology. The airway inflammation is frequently mediated by Th2
lymphocytes, whose cytokine secretion leads to mast cell stimulation,
eosinophilia, leukocytosis, and enhanced B-cell IgE production. Although
various genes have been identified as likely contributors to asthma development, asthma is largely environmentally triggered and has a multifactorial cause. Asthma is extremely common, especially in poor, urban
environments. Asthma is the third most common reason for pediatric
hospitalizations.

The goal of this article is to inform readers of the common and uncommon
signs and symptoms of asthma. After completion of this article, readers
should have a firm understanding of the symptoms and presentation
leading to a diagnosis of asthma.

Pulmonary function testing is an important diagnostic modality in the
workup of patients suspected of having asthma. It is also valuable for

monitoring response to treatment in patients initiated and sustained on asthma therapy, and for assessing patients with symptoms suggestive of an asthma exacerbation. Spirometry is the most useful test in patients suspected of having asthma, and can easily be performed and interpreted in the otolaryngology office with readily available, inexpensive equipment. Pulmonary function testing should be considered for use in all otolaryngology patients with significant rhinitis and in those suspected of having lower respiratory disease.

energy to airways by a catheter-directed expandable basket. The airways of the lower and upper lobes are treated in 3 separate sessions spaced 3 weeks apart. The therapy targets airway smooth muscle, with studies showing a decrease in airway smooth muscle after bronchial thermoplasty therapy. After therapy, an improvement in quality of life and decrease in asthma exacerbations can be expected. Adverse events can occur with bronchial thermoplasty and careful patient selection is critical to ensure benefits outweigh the potential risks.

Measuring fractional exhaled nitric oxide (FeNO) is a relatively new option for assessing allergic inflammation in the lungs. Clinical management of asthma is challenging, and measuring exhaled nitric oxide can provide another type of data to assist in meeting this challenge. FeNO is easy to perform, and the equipment is not forbiddingly expensive. FeNO provides a complement to traditional measures of asthma control and can help guide diagnostic and treatment choices. This article explains what it is, how the measurements are performed, what the norms are, and its use and limitations in the management of asthma.

Vitamin D (vitD3) deficiency occurs frequently and has profound effects on health, especially asthma. This article examines how current knowledge of vitD3 actions and the worldwide distribution of vitD3 deficiency influences everyday clinical allergy practice. Within the limits of current knowledge, the article concisely explains the molecular nature of vitD3 actions, reviews key vitD3 research as it applies to clinical care, answers questions about the potential clinical impact of low vitD3 levels, and discusses use and safety of vitD3 supplements.

Asthma has many triggers including rhinosinusitis; allergy; irritants; medications (aspirin in aspirin-exacerbated respiratory disease); and obesity. Paradoxical vocal fold dysfunction mimics asthma and may be present along with asthma. This article reviews each of these triggers, outlining methods of recognizing the trigger and its management. In many patients more than one trigger may be present. Full appreciation of the complexity of these relationships and targeted therapy to the trigger is needed to best care for the patient with asthma.

Exercise-induced bronchoconstriction (EIB) occurs commonly in patients with asthma but also can affect individuals without asthma. EIB is particularly common in populations of athletes. Common symptoms include cough, dyspnea, chest tightness, and wheezing; however, there can be

OTOLARYNGOLOGIC CLINICS
OF NORTH AMERICA

RELATED INTEREST

Immunology and Allergy Clinics, Volume 33, Issue 1, February 2013
Allergic Rhinitis and Chronic Rhinosinusitis: Their Impact on Lower Airways
Ramakrishnan JB, Kingdom TT, Ramakrishnan VR
http://www.sciencedirect.com/science/article/pii/S0889856112001312
Conditions Mimicking Asthma; Eugene M. Choo, MD, *Editor*

**DOWNLOAD
Free App!**

Review Articles
THE CLINICS

NOW AVAILABLE FOR YOUR iPhone and iPad

Preface

Doc, I Can't Breathe!

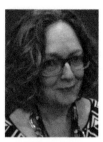

Karen H. Calhoun, MD, FACS, FAAOA
Editor

As otolaryngologists, we are trained to think, first, of surgical airway emergencies requiring tracheostomy or other urgent surgery; second, we think about nasal obstruction. As we provide more allergy care, however, we also need to think of asthma. Here's why:

First: Being able to assess and provide care for asthma is a convenience for our "allergic rhinitis with asthma" patients.

Second: More than that, however, we know that allergic rhinitis patients often have underlying bronchial hyperreactivity[1,2] — and many are unaware of it. It is not uncommon for us to see, say, the patient who has gradually restricted their activity over the years without really thinking about why. Identifying and correcting their bronchial hyperreactivity or asthma can greatly improve their quality of life.

Third: Surveys have shown that a major factor in fatal or near-fatal reactions to testing or subcutaneous immunotherapy is asthma.[3] Selecting our airway-reactive patients for additional pulmonary treatment before testing safeguards our patients — and us!

The articles in this issue are written by experts who are clinically active in asthma care. I think you will find them concise and clear. And I hope they help in your pursuit of excellence in patient care.

Karen H. Calhoun, MD, FACS, FAAOA
Department of Otolaryngology - Head and Neck Surgery
Wexner Medical Center
The Ohio State University College of Medicine
915 Olentangy River Road
Columbus, OH 43212, USA
http://sinusallergy.osu.edu

E-mail address:
karen.calhoun@osumc.edu

Otolaryngol Clin N Am 47 (2014) xiii–xiv
http://dx.doi.org/10.1016/j.otc.2013.10.011
0030-6665/14/$ – see front matter © 2014 Published by Elsevier Inc.

REFERENCES

1. Cirillo I, Ricciardolo FL, Medusei G, et al. Exhaled nitric oxide may predict bronchial hyperreactivity in patients with allergic rhinitis. Int Arch Allergy Immunol 2013;160:332–8.
2. Skiepko R, Zietkowski Z, Tomasiak-Lozowska MM, et al. Bronchial hyperreponsiveness and airway inflammation in patients with seasonal allergy rhinitis. J Investig Allergol Clin Immunol 2011;21:532–9.
3. Bernstein DI, Wanner M, Borish L, et al. Immunotherapy Committee, American Academy of Allergy, Asthma and Immunology. Twelve-year survey of fatal reactions to allergen injections and skin testing: 1990-2001. J Allergy Clin Immunol 2004;113:1129–36.

Why Otolaryngologists and Asthma Are a Good Match
The Allergic Rhinitis-Asthma Connection

Rachel Georgopoulos, MD, John H. Krouse, MD, PhD,
Elina Toskala, MD, PhD*

KEYWORDS

- Asthma • Rhinitis • Allergy • Immunology

KEY POINTS

- In the unified airway model, the nose and the paranasal sinuses through the respiratory bronchi are considered as components of 1 functional unit.
- Rhinitis and asthma are linked epidemiologically and pathophysiologically.
- Rhinitis is not only associated with but is a risk factor for the development of asthma.
- Atopy/allergy and disease severity are important factors affecting the association between rhinitis and asthma.
- Hygiene hypothesis suggests that a lack of microbial exposures as a child may result in modification of immunity toward T helper 2 (Th_2) skewing and the increased risk for asthma and other atopic diseases.
- Proper management of allergic rhinitis can concomitantly allow better asthma control.
- In evaluating and treating patients with rhinitis, the diagnosis of asthma should be considered.
- It is important that physicians managing rhinitis/rhinosinusitis become familiar with the diagnosis and management of asthma.

INTRODUCTION

Although rhinitis and asthma are frequently comorbid conditions, physicians managing patients with rhinitis and or rhinosinusitis have traditionally not taken part in the diagnosis or management of asthma. Rhinitis, sinusitis, and asthma are linked both epidemiologically and pathophysiologically and thus the nose through the paranasal sinuses to the distal bronchioles should not be thought of as separate entities but rather constituents of 1 functional unit. This unit is referred to as the unified airway model.[1-3] Rhinitis is not only associated with but is a risk factor for the development

Department of Otolaryngology, Temple University Health System, 3509 North Broad Street, Philadelphia, PA 19140-4105, USA
* Corresponding author.
E-mail address: elina.toskala@tuhs.temple.edu

Otolaryngol Clin N Am 47 (2014) 1–12
http://dx.doi.org/10.1016/j.otc.2013.08.016
0030-6665/14/$ – see front matter © 2014 Elsevier Inc. All rights reserved.

Abbreviations	
AR	Allergic rhinitis
BHR	Bronchial hyperresponsiveness
CGRP	Calcitonin gene-related peptide
ICS	Inhaled corticosteroids
LABA	Long-acting β2-agonists
RSV	Respiratory syncytial virus
SABAs	Short-acting bronchodilators

of asthma.[4–11] Although both allergic and nonallergic forms of rhinitis are associated with asthma, the association between asthma and allergic rhinitis (AR) is even stronger.[4,11] The use of allergen-directed immunotherapy in young children with allergic rhinitis has been shown to prevent the development of asthma in later life.[12–14] Irritants and allergens presented at one portion of the airway have distal effects. It is thought that the upper and lower airways communicate through a complex interaction of inflammatory mediators and the autonomic system. Furthermore, disease severities in rhinitis and asthma often parallel each other.[4,15] Adequate treatment of allergic rhinitis can allow better asthma control and, in some situations, may even prevent the development of asthma.[16–20] With the substantial evidence to support the link between upper and lower airway disease it is imperative that physicians who manage patients with rhinitis and sinusitis become familiar with the diagnosis and management of asthma.

AR AND ASTHMA DEFINED

AR is defined as a symptomatic immunoglobulin E (IgE)–mediated inflammation of the nasal mucosa.[9] Symptoms of rhinitis are reversible and include nasal congestion/obstruction, rhinorrhea, sneezing, pruritus, postnasal drip, chronic cough, throat clearing, and conjunctivitis.[9,21] Rhinitis is categorized, based on duration of symptoms and by the disease's impact on quality of life, as intermittent or persistent mild or moderate to severe (**Table 1**).[9]

Asthma is a chronic inflammatory disorder of the airways that results in reversible airway obstruction and bronchial hyperresponsiveness (BHR) to a variety of stimuli. Inflammatory mediators and mainly mast cells, eosinophils, T lymphocytes, neutrophils, and epithelial cells are known to play an important role in this process. In advanced cases, airway remodeling can occur, with irreversible injury to the pulmonary mucosa. The airway inflammation and subsequent airway obstruction experienced by these individuals can result in symptoms of wheezing, breathlessness, chest tightness, and coughing.[22,23]

Although the focus of asthma pathophysiology was once on the hyperresponsiveness of the airways, it is now known that inflammation is the driving mechanism, with the increased bronchial reactivity being caused by this inflammatory state. This concept is important to understanding the pathophysiology and treatment of asthmatics.

EPIDEMIOLOGY
Asthma-Rhinitis Link

AR and asthma affect about 30% and 7% to 8% of people respectively.[6,24,25] Between 75% and 80% of atopic and nonatopic individuals with asthma have rhinitis.[9] Between 10% and 40% of individuals with rhinitis have asthma.[26] Not only are rhinitis and asthma associated but rhinitis is a risk factor for the development of asthma. Twenty percent of individuals with rhinitis go on to develop asthma later in life. Studies suggest

Table 1 Classification of allergic rhinitis	
Intermittent	Symptoms present for: • Less than 4 d/wk • Or for less than 4 wk/y
Persistent	Symptoms present for: • More than 4 d/wk • Or for more than 4 wk/y
Mild	Patient does not experience: • Sleep disturbance • Impairment of daily activities, leisure, and/or sport • Impairment of school or work • Troublesome symptoms
Moderate to severe	Patient experiences 1 or more of the following: • Sleep disturbance • Impairment of daily activities, leisure, and/or sport • Impairment of school or work • Troublesome symptoms

Adapted from Bousquet J, Van Cauwenberge P, Khaltaev N, ARIA Workshop Group, World Health Organization. Allergic rhinitis and its impact on asthma. J Allergy Clin Immunol 2001;108(5):147–336; with permission.

that individuals with rhinitis have a 3-fold increased risk for the development of asthma.[4,5,7] Rhinitis often precedes the development of asthma.

This association is influenced by a variety of factors. The development of atopy in early childhood, before 6 years of age, is an important risk factor for the development of BHR in late childhood.[27] However, although early sensitization to inhalant allergens is a known risk factor for the development of atopic disease later in life, only about 25% of individuals sensitized to one or more inhalant allergen go on to develop asthma.[28] Among individuals with AR and atopy the type of protein to which the individual is sensitized correlates with differing propensities for development of asthma. Individuals sensitized to perennial allergens have a significantly higher likelihood for developing asthma than individuals sensitized to seasonal allergens.[11,29] In a study by Linneberg and colleagues,[11] compared with their nonallergic counterparts, individuals sensitized to pollen, a seasonal allergen, had a 10-fold increased risk for developing asthma, whereas those who were sensitized to dust mite, a perennial allergen, had a 50-fold increased risk for developing asthma.

Genetics

In addition, there seems to be a genetic predilection to the development of these diseases. In a study in northern Sweden, a family history of atopic rhinitis and atopic asthma increased the risk of developing those conditions up to 6-fold and 4-fold respectively.[30]

Geography

Significant geographic variability exists in reference to the prevalence of allergic respiratory diseases. Dahl and colleagues[31] performed a study looking at the prevalence of patient-reported allergic respiratory disorders in 10 European countries. Spain had a significantly lower prevalence and Italy a significantly higher prevalence of allergic respiratory disorder compared with other European countries: 11.7% and 33.6%, respectively (**Table 2**).[31]

Table 2	
Prevalence of allergic respiratory disorder in 10 European countries	
Country	Prevalence (%)[a]
Italy	33.6
Norway	26.8
Sweden	26.8
United Kingdom	26.2
Finland	26.0
The Netherlands	24.2
Germany	23.5
Denmark	20.6
Austria	15.9
Spain	11.7

[a] Nationally balanced prevalence % weighted against size of national population.
Adapted from Dahl R, Andersen PS, Chivato T, et al. National prevalence of respiratory allergic disorders. Respir Med 2004;98(5):398–403; with permission.

Disease Severity

Disease severity also has an important influence on this association. Individuals with severe, persistent forms of rhinitis are more likely to have symptomatic asthma than individuals with intermittent forms of rhinitis.[4,15] Patients with asthma and severe rhinitis experience a higher rate of nighttime awakenings and increased absences from work than asthmatics with less severe rhinitis.[15]

Environmental Factors Beyond Allergens

In addition to allergens, there are a variety of environmental factors that have been implicated in the development of asthma. As an example, there is a known association between respiratory symptoms such as dyspnea on exertion, breathlessness, and cough with air pollution.[32] Furthermore, exposure to moisture damage at work or at home and other causes of occupational rhinitis are well-studied risk factors.[33–35] The risk of asthma has been shown to be as high as 7 times that of controls among farmers with occupational rhinitis.[34] Although further studies need to be performed, reduced exposure to known occupational triggers for rhinitis is important not only for symptom management but also for the potential prevention of occupational asthma. Furthermore, tobacco smoke, drugs such as aspirin, obesity, and viral infections such as respiratory syncytial virus are known risk factors for the development of asthma.[36–40]

Allergens and/or irritants cause local inflammation in the nasal mucosa that leads to an increased ability for inhaled irritants to get to the distal bronchioles by disrupting the filtering capabilities of the nose, which results in the inhalation of unfiltered irritants into the distal airways and subsequently pulmonary symptoms. However, even in the absence of a local response, allergens/irritants presented to an isolated portion of the respiratory system exert distal effects.

PATHOPHYSIOLOGY

Two mechanisms have been proposed to explain the communication between the nasal and bronchial mucosa:

1. Inflammatory crosstalk in which local irritation leads to upregulation of a variety of inflammatory mediators at a distal site within the respiratory tract[41–43]

2. Neurogenic reflexes, in which neuronal stimulation in the nose can result in the release of cholinergic neurotransmitters and subsequent contraction of the bronchial smooth muscle[44,45]

Inflammatory Response

A series of studies were performed by Braunstahl and colleagues[41–43] in which antigen placed in the nose resulted in upregulation of inflammatory mediators at the distal bronchi, and inoculation of an antigen into the bronchi using a bronchoscope resulted in upregulation of inflammatory mediators in the nose. The upregulation of inflammatory mediators at a site distal to inoculation suggests an inflammatory crosstalk between the upper and lower airway systems. Bronchoconstriction results from the interaction between resident inflammatory cells, such as mast cells and alveolar macrophages, with upregulated inflammatory mediators such as eosinophils, lymphocytes, neutrophils, and basophils. Mediators such as histamine, leukotrienes, prostaglandin D_2, and platelet-activating factor, are subsequently released and act on bronchial smooth muscle to cause muscle contraction.[22,46]

Autonomic Response

Either by direct activation of the vagus nerve or via secondary activation of the parasympathetic system, neuroregulatory mechanisms act at the level of the bronchial smooth muscle to result in bronchoconstriction. Neuromediators such as substance P and calcitonin gene-related peptide, affect the release of histamine and bradykinin. These mediators work at the vascular epithelium to cause an unrestricted passage of proteins and fluid. In addition, cholinergic neurotransmitters cause contraction of the bronchial smooth muscle.[46–50] Moreover, mucus plugging from excessive mucus production further contributes to airflow obstruction.[46]

Histopathology

The nose, paranasal sinuses, trachea, and primary and secondary bronchi are all lined by a pseudostratified ciliated columnar epithelium.[1] The inflammatory cell profile in the nasal mucosa of patients with AR is similar to that seen in the bronchial mucosa of patients with atopic asthma, with both having an increased infiltration of mainly eosinophils, as well as a variety of other cytokines.[51,52]

Unlike the lower respiratory tract, the nasal passages have an extensive vascular system with subepithelial capillaries, arteries, and venous and cavernous sinusoids.[9] Vessel engorgement results in symptomatic nasal obstruction, which is one of the characteristic features of rhinitis. In contrast, the trachea through the respiratory bronchi is lined by smooth muscle. It is the contraction of this smooth muscle system either through the inflammatory or neuroregulatory mechanisms discussed earlier that causes the acute, reversible airway obstruction that is the pathognomonic feature of asthma.

T helper 2 (Th_2) cells are responsible for allergic inflammation. Interleukin (IL)-4, IL-5, and IL-13, along with other inflammatory mediators and chemokines, result in the transendothelial migration and activation of eosinophils.[46,53–56] In addition, endothelial adhesion proteins intercellular adhesion molecule-1 and vascular cell adhesion molecule-1 assist in the migration of neutrophils, lymphocytes, and eosinophils from the intravascular space into the airway. Mast cell degranulation and histamine release lead to the production of leukotrienes. Eosinophils present in the inflamed tissue causes the release of toxic basic proteins, which leads to epithelial damage and airflow obstruction.[46] This processes results in the characteristic histologic features of mucosal edema, submucosal gland and bronchial smooth muscle hypertrophy, mucus hypersecretion, and basement membrane thickening and fibrosis seen in asthma.[46,57–59]

Chronic inflammation in asthmatics can result in airway remodeling. Remodeling is a process in which tissue injury and subsequent repair leads to mucosal edema, submucosal gland and bronchial smooth muscle hypertrophy, mucus gland and goblet cell hyperplasia, angiogenesis, collagen deposition, basement membrane thickening, and subepithelial fibrosis in the lamina reticularis.[46,57–59] Although similar finding are seen in patients with chronic rhinosinusitis, remodeling has not been well shown in patients with allergic rhinitis. Further, the reticular basement membrane thickening is not as pronounced in nasal epithelium in rhinitis as it is in the bronchial epithelium in patients with asthma.[60]

ASTHMA AND ATOPY

There are 2 categories of T lymphocytes, Th_1 and Th_2, with atopic patients having a skewed predilection for the Th_2 phenotype.[61–63] Th_2 cells lead to the production of IgE antibodies and the upregulation of eosinophils, and various interleukins such as IL-4, IL-5, and IL-13.[18,46,54–56,61] This process is sustained by cytokines such as IL-4 that work through positive feedback mechanisms to perpetuate the Th_2 pathway and downregulate Th_1 cells.[62]

Many theories have been proposed to explain the increased prevalence of asthma, particularly in the pediatric population. One theory is referred to as the hygiene hypothesis. In this model, the increased predilection for the Th_2 cytokine response is attributed to a decreased microbial exposure in the postnatal period.[61] Microbial exposure early in life is a known stimulus for normal Th_1 maturation.[64] With improvements in management and prevention of infection through advancements in antibiotics, vaccination, and various public health measures, there has been a decreased microbial stimulus for the Th_1 phenotype. This theory has been supported by multiple studies. Children with increased exposure to infection early in life have fewer symptoms of BHR.[65] In addition, it has been shown that atopy is less prevalent among children raised in large families and or on farms.

DIAGNOSIS

The work-up and evaluation of patients with rhinitis and or asthma should include a thorough assessment of both the upper and lower airways. In light of the significant association with allergy, it is important to inquire about presence of atopic disease; seasonality of symptoms; known triggers; or locations, such as work, in which symptoms worsen; and family history of atopic disease. In addition, it is important to ask whether allergy or pulmonary function testing has been performed and whether the patient has been or is on inhaled, topical, or oral medications for upper or lower airway disease. Along with asking about nasal symptoms such as nasal congestion/obstruction, hyposmia/anosmia, sneezing, postnasal drip, throat clearing, and chronic cough, it is important to ask about symptoms of shortness of breath with exercise, prolonged cough after viral infections, and nighttime cough. However, patients with cough-variant asthma may not present with the classic asthma symptoms such as wheezing.

Physical examination in these patients should include a thorough head and neck examination with particular attention to signs of atopy. Some examples include darkening of the skin beneath the eyes, referred to as allergic shiners, fine lines of the eyelids, referred to as Dennie lines, and a horizontal crease across the lower bridge of the nose referred to as the allergic salute.[66] Conjunctival erythema may also be appreciated. Rhinoscopy is a valuable tool in the evaluation of patients with AR and or asthma. Rigid or flexible endoscopy is preferred but in their absence an otoscope can be placed in the nares. Attention should be paid to the appearance of the nasal mucosa. In cases of AR the nasal mucosa is often boggy and pale, whereas in cases of nonallergic rhinitis the mucosa is often erythematous and inflamed. The quality of nasal secretion, position of the nasal septum, and/or the presence of polyps should also be noted. Examination of the oropharynx in patients with AR may reveal irregularities of the posterior pharynx, referred to as cobblestoning, which is often seen in patients with atopy. Otoscopic examination may reveal signs of effusion. The skin should be examined for signs of eczema and/or dermatitis, which can be present in atopic patients. In addition, a pulmonary examination should be performed. Auscultation may reveal prolonged forced exhalation and expiratory wheezes. Percussion of the lungs may reveal hyper-resonant breath sounds as a result of air trapping.[1]

A diagnosis of asthma is based on the presence of a variety of symptoms with episodic and at least partially reversible airway obstruction.[22] Although symptoms of breathlessness, cough, recurrent wheezing, and/or chest tightness are common in asthma, they are not diagnostic. Objective measures of pulmonary function can help delineate asthma from a variety of other pulmonary disorders including restrictive airway diseases, other obstructive pulmonary diseases, vocal fold dysfunction, and central airway obstruction. There are a variety of tests used to assess pulmonary function, including lung volumes, spirometry, flow volume loops, diffusion capacity, and body plethysmography.[1]

In patients with allergic rhinitis, allergy testing with either skin prick test or allergen-specific IgE (radioallergosorbent testing [RAST]) should be performed. Although test results take longer with RAST, it is useful in patients with dermographism, dermatitis, and in cases in which antihistamines cannot be discontinued.[67]

TREATMENT

In patients with known IgE-mediated sensitization, avoidance of sensitized allergens has been shown to improve rhinitis and asthma control and is therefore recommended in all atopic patients.[68]

Treatment of rhinitis has been shown to improve asthma control.[16,17,53,69,70] Intranasal corticosteroids are often used as first-line agents in the management of AR. Not only have intranasal corticosteroids been found to be efficacious in the management of moderate to severe rhinitis they have also been shown to reduce BHR and improve asthma symptoms.[16,17]

At present, there are 2 classes of medications used in the management of asthmatics, referred to as controller and reliever medications.[71]

- Controller medications such as corticosteroids and immunomodulators are used to treat the underlying inflammatory process in an attempt to prevent adverse outcomes.
- Reliever or rescue medications, including short-acting bronchodilators and inhaled anticholinergics, are used to treat the acute symptoms of bronchoconstriction including dyspnea, wheezing, and cough.

Inhaled corticosteroids (ICSs) are the first-line controller therapy used in the treatment of asthma.[22] Not only has ICS been shown to decrease airway inflammation and BHR but it has also been shown to improve nasal symptoms and pulmonary function scores, reduce the frequency and severity of asthma exacerbations, and reduce asthma-related mortality.[71] Long-acting β2-agonists (LABA) are used in combination with ICSs for long-term control and prevention in moderate or severe persistent asthma.

LABAs are not used as a monotherapy because they do not have efficacy as an antiin-flammatory agent and are associated with increased risk of asthma-related deaths.[69]

The use of both intranasal and inhaled steroids has been shown to reduce the number of emergency department visits, as well as the number of asthma-related work absences and asthma-related episodes of nighttime awakening.[16]

Systemic corticosteroids have been efficacious in the management of both rhinitis and asthma but, as a result of their side effect profile, systemic corticosteroid therapy is only used in severe refractory cases.

Immunomodulators such as omalizumab, a monoclonal anti-IgE antibody, has shown efficacy in both the treatment of asthma and allergic rhinitis but its use is limited because of significantly high costs.[22,72,73]

AR often precedes the development of asthma, and therefore early and aggressive management of AR should be used in order to potentially prevent the development of asthma in later life. Immunotherapy to sensitized allergens in patients with AR has shown promising results in terms of reduced symptoms, reduced need for medication, and potential prevention of asthma.[12]

SUMMARY

Consideration of the unified airway model when managing patients with rhinitis and or asthma allows a more comprehensive care plan and therefore improved patient outcomes. Asthma is clearly linked to rhinitis both epidemiologically and biologically, and this association is even stronger in individuals with atopy. Rhinitis is not only associated with but is a risk factor for the development of asthma.[4–10] As a result, physicians managing rhinitis may be the first health care providers able to identify early signs of asthma. Management of rhinitis has been shown to improve asthma control. Early and aggressive treatment of allergic rhinitis may prevent the development of asthma. In patients with allergic rhinitis that is not sufficiently controlled by allergy medication, allergen-directed immunotherapy should be considered.

REFERENCES

1. Krouse JH, Brown RW, Fineman SM, et al. Asthma and the unified airway. Otolaryngol Head Neck Surg 2007;136(5):S75–106.
2. Krouse JH. Allergy and chronic rhinosinusitis. Otolaryngol Clin North Am 2005; 38:1257–66.
3. Krouse JH. The unified airway–conceptual framework. Otolaryngol Clin North Am 2008;41:257–66.
4. Guerra S, Sherrill DL, Martinez FD, et al. Rhinitis as an independent risk factor for adult-onset asthma. J Allergy Clin Immunol 2002;109:419–25.
5. Corren J. Allergic rhinitis and asthma: how important is the link? J Allergy Clin Immunol 1997;99:S781–6.
6. Blomme K, Tomassen P, Lapeere H. Prevalence of allergic sensitization versus allergic rhinitis symptoms in an unselected population. Int Arch Allergy Immunol 2013;160(2):200–7.
7. Settipane RJ, Hagy GW, Settipane GA. Long-term risk factors for developing asthma and allergic rhinitis: a 23-year follow-up of college students. Allergy Proc 1994;15:21–5.
8. Leynaert B, Bousquet J, Neukirch C, et al. Perennial rhinitis: an independent risk factor for asthma in nonatopic subjects: results from the European Community Respiratory Health Survey. J Allergy Clin Immunol 1999;104(2):301–4.

9. Bousquet J, Van Cauwenberge P, Khaltaev N, ARIA Workshop Group, World Health Organization. Allergic rhinitis and its impact on asthma. J Allergy Clin Immunol 2001;108(5):147–336.

10. Meltzer EO, Hamilos DL, Hadley JA, et al. Rhinosinusitis: establishing definitions for clinical research and patient care. Otolaryngol Head Neck Surg 2004;131(6): S1–62.

11. Linneberg A, Henrick Nielsen N, Frolund L, et al. The link between allergic rhinitis and asthma: a prospective, population-based study, the Copenhagen Allergy Study. Allergy 2002;57:1048–52.

12. Möller C, Dreborg S, Ferdousi HA, et al. Pollen immunotherapy reduces the development of asthma in children with seasonal rhino-conjunctivitis (the PAT study). J Allergy Clin Immunol 2002;109(2):251–6.

13. Johnstone DE, Dutton A. The value of hyposensitization therapy for bronchial asthma in children–A 14 year study. Pediatrics 1968;42:793–802.

14. Jacobsen L, Nuchel Petersen B, Wihl HA, et al. Immunotherapy with partially purified and standardized tree pollen extracts. IV: results from long-term (6 year) follow-up. Allergy 1997;52:914–20.

15. Huse DM, Harte SC, Russel MW, et al. Allergic rhinitis may worsen asthma symptoms in children: the international Asthma Outcomes registry. Am J Respir Crit Care Med 1996;153:A860.

16. Stelmach R, do Patrocinio T Nunes M, Ribeiro M, et al. Effect of treating allergic rhinitis with corticosteroids in patients with mild-to-moderate persistent asthma. Chest 2005;128(5):3140–7.

17. Watson WT, Becker AB, Simons FE. Treatment of allergic rhinitis with intranasal corticosteroids in patients with mild asthma: effect on lower airway responsiveness. J Allergy Clin Immunol 1993;91:97–101.

18. Jani A, Hamilos DL. Current thinking on the relationship between rhinosinusitis and asthma. J Asthma 2005;42(1):1–7.

19. Lund V. The effect of sinonasal surgery on asthma. Allergy 1999;57:141–5.

20. Aubier M, Neukirch C, Peiffer C, et al. Effect of cetirizine on bronchial hyperresponsiveness in patients with seasonal allergic rhinitis and asthma. Allergy 2001; 56:35–42.

21. Corey JP, Gungor A, Karnell M. Allergy for the laryngologist. Otolaryngol Clin North Am 1998;31(1):189–205.

22. National Heart, Lung, and Blood Institute: National Institute of Health; U.S. Department of Health and Human services: Expert panel report 3: guidelines for the diagnosis and management of asthma. NIH publication no. 07–4051, National Institutes of Health; National Heart, Lung, and Blood Institute; Bethesda (MD). 2007. Available at: http://www.nhlbi.nih.gov.libproxy.temple.edu/guidelines/asthma. Accessed March, 2013.

23. Expert panel report: guidelines for the diagnosis and management of asthma (EPR 1991). Bethesda (MD): US Department of Health and Human Services; National Institutes of Health; National Heart, Lung, and Blood Institute; National Asthma Education and Prevention Program; 1991.

24. Akinbami LJ. Asthma prevalence, health care use, and mortality: United States, 2005–2009. Natl Health Stat Report 2011;(32):1–16.

25. Schiller JS, Lucas JW, Peregoy JA. Summary health statistics for U.S. adults: National Health Interview Survey, 2011. National Center for Health Statistics. US Department of Health and Human Services Centers for Disease Control and Prevention. Vital Health Stat 2012;(252):1–207.

26. Bousquet J, Khaltaev N, Cruz AA, et al. Allergic Rhinitis and its Impact on Asthma (ARIA) 2008 update (in collaboration with the World Health Organization. GA(2)LEN and AllerGen). Allergy 2008;63(86):8–160.
27. Peat JK, Salome CM, Woolcock AJ. Longitudinal changes in atopy during a 4-year period: relation to bronchial hyperresponsiveness and respiratory symptoms in a population sample of Australian schoolchildren. J Allergy Clin Immunol 1990;85:65–74.
28. Jones C, Holt P. Immunopathology of allergy and asthma in childhood. Am J Respir Crit Care Med 2000;162:S36–9.
29. Prieto J, Gutierrez V, Berto JM, et al. Sensitivity and maximal response to methacholine in perennial and seasonal allergic rhinitis. Clin Exp Allergy 1996;26:61–7.
30. Lundback B. Epidemiology of rhinitis and asthma. Clin Exp Allergy 1998;2:3–10.
31. Dahl R, Andersen PS, Chivato T, et al. National prevalence of respiratory allergic disorders. Respir Med 2004;98(5):398–403.
32. Zemp E, Elsasser S, Schindler C, et al. Long term ambient air pollution and respiratory symptoms in adults (SAPALDIA Study). Am J Respir Crit Care Med 1999;159:1257–66.
33. Karvala K, Toskala E, Luukkonen R. New-onset adult asthma in relation to damp and moldy workplaces. Int Arch Occup Environ Health 2010;83(8):855–65.
34. Karjalainen A, Martikainen T, Klaukka T, et al. Risk of asthma among Finnish patients with occupational rhinitis. chest 2003;123:283–8.
35. Ameille J, Hamelin K, Andujar P, et al. Occupational asthma and occupational rhinitis: the united airways disease model revisited. Occup Environ Med 2013; 70:471–5.
36. Strachan DP, Cook DG. Health effects of passive smoking. 6. Parental smoking and childhood asthma: longitudinal and case control studies. Thorax 1998; 53(3):204–12.
37. Eisner MD, Yelin EH, Henke J, et al. Environmental tobacco smoke and adult asthma. The impact of changing exposure status on health outcomes. Am J Respir Crit Care Med 1998;158:170–5.
38. Ford ES. The epidemiology of obesity and asthma. J Allergy Clin Immunol 2005; 115(5):897–909.
39. Stein RT, Sherrill D, Morgan WJ, et al. Respiratory syncytial virus in early life and risk of wheeze and allergy by age 13 years. Lancet 1999;354(9178):541–5.
40. Johnston SL, Pattemore PK, Sanderson G, et al. Community study of role of viral infections in exacerbations of asthma in 9–11 year old children. BMJ 1995; 310(6989):1225–9.
41. Braunstahl GJ, Kleinjan A, Overbeek SE, et al. Segmental bronchial provocation induces nasal inflammation in allergic rhinitis patients. Am J Respir Crit Care Med 2000;161:2051–7.
42. Braunstahl GJ, Overbeek SE, Kleinjan A, et al. Nasal allergen provocation induces adhesion molecule expression and tissue eosinophila in upper and lower airways. J Allergy Clin Immunol 2001;107(3):469–76.
43. Braunstahl GJ, Overbeek SE, Fokkens WJ, et al. Segmental bronchoprovocation in allergic rhinitis patients affects mast cell and basophil numbers in nasal and bronchial mucosa. Am J Respir Crit Care Med 2001;164:858–65.
44. Fontanari P, Burnet H, Zatarra-Hartmann MC, et al. Changes in airway resistance induced by nasal inhalation of cold dry, dry, or moist air in normal individuals. J Appl Physiol 1996;81(4):1739–43.
45. Sarin S, Undem B, Sanico A, et al. The role of the nervous system in rhinitis. J Allergy Clin Immunol 2006;118(5):999–1014.

46. Lemanske RF, Busse WW. Asthma. J Allergy Clin Immunol 2003;111(2):502–19.
47. Erjavec F, Lembeck F, Florjanc-Irman T, et al. Release of histamine by substance P. Naunyn Schmiedebergs Arch Pharmacol 1981;317:67–70.
48. Piotrowski W, Foreman JC. Some effects of calcitonin gene-related peptide in human skin and on histamine release. Br J Dermatol 1986;114(1):37–46.
49. Mehta D, Malik AB. Signaling mechanisms regulating endothelial permeability. Physiol Rev 2006;86(1):279–367.
50. Canning BJ. Reflex regulation of airway smooth muscle tone. J Appl Phys 2006; 101(3):971–85.
51. Togias A. Rhinitis and asthma: evidence for respiratory system integration. J Allergy Clin Immunol 2003;111(6):1171–83.
52. Calderon M, Losewicz S, Prior A, et al. Lymphocyte infiltration and thickness of the nasal mucous membrane in perennial and seasonal allergic rhinitis. J Allergy Clin Immunol 1994;93:635–43.
53. Shturman-Ellstein R, Zeballos RJ, Buckley JM, et al. The beneficial effect of nasal breathing on exercise-induced bronchoconstriction. Am Rev Respir Dis 1978;118(1):65–73.
54. Hamilos D. Chronic sinusitis. J Allergy Clin Immunol 2000;106:213–27.
55. Bachert C, Vignola AM, Gevaert P, et al. Allergic rhinitis, rhinosinusitis, and asthma: one airway disease. Immunol Allergy Clin North Am 2004;24(1):19–43.
56. Alam R, Stafford RA, Forsythe P, et al. RANTES is a chemotactic and activating factor for human eosinophils. J Immunol 1993;150(8):3442–8.
57. Dunnill MS. The pathology of asthma with special reference to changes in the bronchial mucosa. J Clin Pathol 1960;13:27–33.
58. Dunnill MS, Massarella GR, Anderson JA. A comparison of the quantitative anatomy of the bronchi in normal subjects in status asthmaticus in chronic bronchitis, and in emphysema. Thorax 1969;24(2):176–9.
59. Kay AB. Asthma and inflammation. J Allergy Clin Immunol 1991;87(5):893–910.
60. Bousquet J, Jacquot W, Vignola M, et al. Allergic rhinitis: a disease remodeling the upper airways? J Allergy Clin Immunol 2004;113:43–9.
61. Romagnani S. Human TH1 and TH2 subsets: doubt no more. Immunol Today 1991;12(8):256–7.
62. Maddox L, Schwartz DA. The pathophysiology of asthma. Annu Rev Med 2002; 53:477–98.
63. Abbas AK, Murphy KM, Sher A. Functional diversity of helper T lymphocytes. Nature 1996;383:787–93.
64. Holt PG, Macaubas C. Development of long-term tolerance versus sensitisation to environmental allergens during the perinatal period. Curr Opin Immunol 1997; 9:782–7.
65. Ball TM, Castro-Rodriquez JA, Griffin KA, et al. Siblings, day-care attendance, and the risk of asthma and wheezing during childhood. N Engl J Med 2000; 343:538–43.
66. Fornadley JA, Corey JP, Osguthorpe JD, et al. Allergic rhinitis: clinical practice guideline. Committee on Practice Standards, American Academy of Otolaryngic Allergy. Otolaryngol Head Neck Surg 1996;115(1):115–22.
67. Greiner AN, Hellings PW, Rotiroti G. Allergic rhinitis. Lancet 2012;378(9809):2112–22.
68. Bush RK. The use of anti-IgE in the treatment of allergic asthma. Med Clin North Am 2002;86:1113–29.
69. Taramarcaz P, Gibson PG. Intranasal corticosteroids for asthma control in people with coexisting asthma and rhinitis. Cochrane Database Syst Rev 2003;(4):CD003570.

70. Dejima K, Hama T, Miyazaki M, et al. A clinical study of endoscopic sinus surgery for sinusitis in patients with bronchial asthma. Allerg Immunol 2005; 138(2):97–104.
71. Global initiative for asthma: global strategy for asthma management and prevention. 2013. Available at: www.ginasthma.org. Accessed April 9, 2013.
72. Dimov VV, Casale TB. Immunomodulators for asthma. Allergy Asthma Immunol Res 2010;2(4):228–34.
73. Nelson HS, Weiss ST, Bleeker ER, et al. The Salmeterol Multicenter Asthma Research Trial: a comparison of usual pharmacotherapy for asthma or usual pharmacotherapy plus salmeterol. Chest 2006;129(5):15–26.

What is Asthma? Pathophysiology, Demographics, and Health Care Costs

Jonathan Maslan, MD, James W. Mims, MD*

KEYWORDS

- Asthma • Pathogenesis • Pathophysiology • Epidemiology • Demographics • Costs

KEY POINTS

- Cardinal asthma symptoms are shortness of breath, cough, chest tightness, and/or wheezing.
- Symptoms arise from airway inflammation, which leads to airway edema, remodeling, and hyperresponsiveness.
- The inflammation in asthma is mediated by multiple cell types including mast cells, eosinophils, lymphocytes, macrophages, neutrophils, and epithelial cells, and there is a predominantly Th2 milieu.
- The cause of asthma is a multifactorial. Active research in asthma genetics has replicated genes that likely play a role in asthma development, but phenotype expression is profoundly affected by environmental triggers.
- Roughly 8% of the US population has asthma and it is the third leading cause of hospitalization in children, accounting for roughly $56 billion per year in direct costs and lost productivity.

WHAT IS ASTHMA?

Asthma is a chronic inflammatory disorder characterized by airway obstruction and hyperresponsiveness. The medical term "asthma," which derives from the Greek for "panting," was named by Hippocrates around 400 BC. Sir William Osler described asthma in his *Principles and Practice of Medicine* in the early 20th century as "swelling of the nasal or respiratory mucous membrane, increased secretion, and…spasm of the bronchial muscles with dyspnea, chiefly expiratory." Of its treatment, he said, "Ordinary tobacco cigarettes are sometimes helpful."[1] (This position is no longer considered true.) Many decades later, it is now understood that asthma is a complex disease

Wake Forest School of Medicine, Medical Center Boulevard, Winston-Salem, NC 27157, USA
* Corresponding author. Department of Otolaryngology, Wake Forest School of Medicine, Medical Center Boulevard, Winston-Salem, NC 27157.
E-mail address: wmims@wakehealth.edu

Otolaryngol Clin N Am 47 (2014) 13–22
http://dx.doi.org/10.1016/j.otc.2013.09.010
0030-6665/14/$ – see front matter © 2014 Elsevier Inc. All rights reserved.

of airway inflammation characterized by airway edema, remodeling, and hyperrespon-siveness. Asthma exacerbations are characterized by progressively worsening short-ness of breath, cough, chest tightness, and/or wheezing. Under this umbrella of clinical symptoms, there is a very sophisticated interplay between underlying geno-types and environmental triggers that is only partially understood. This leads to a broad array of variable disease phenotypes and manifestations. Asthma is increas-ingly recognized as a syndrome, rather than an illness.[2]

Diagnosis

The diagnosis of asthma is made when episodic symptoms of airflow obstruction or airway hyperresponsiveness are present, airflow obstruction is partially reversible, and alternative diagnoses are excluded.[3] In addition to a good medical history and physical examination, spirometry is needed to demonstrate obstruction and assess reversibility.[3] Reversibility is determined by an increase in forced expiratory volume in 1 second (FEV_1) of greater than or equal to 12% from baseline or an increase greater than or equal to 10% of predicted FEV_1 after inhalation of a short-acting β_2-agonist.[3] The National Institutes of Health Guidelines for the Diagnosis and Management of Asthma recommend considering a diagnosis of asthma when certain key indicators are present (**Table 1**). The key indicators consist of specific symptoms, physical ex-amination findings, and modifying factors and environmental exposures. There is a great deal of overlap between asthma symptoms and other disorders of the respira-tory tract. The differential diagnosis for asthma symptoms includes allergic rhinitis or sinusitis, foreign body, aspiration, gastroesophageal reflux, laryngotracheomalacia, vocal cord dysfunction, bronchiolitis, chronic obstructive pulmonary disease, and cystic fibrosis, among other conditions.[3] Recurrent cough and wheezing should al-ways alert practitioners to the possibility of asthma.

Asthma can be intermittent or persistent, and it can present with acute flares or chronic symptoms. Asthma severity is measured by objective measures of lung func-tion (ie, spirometry or peak flow meter) and by symptoms. Measures of impairment include nighttime awakenings, need for short-acting bronchodilators, work or school

Table 1 Key indicators in asthma		
Symptoms	**Physical Examination Findings**	**Modifying Factors**
Wheezing (recurrent)	Thoracic hyperexpansion	Exercise
Cough, worse at night	Wheezing during normal breathing	Viral infection
Difficulty breathing (recurrent)	Prolonged phase of forced exhalation	Animals with fur or hair
Chest tightness (recurrent)	Rhinorrhea	Dust mites
	Nasal polyps	Mold
	Atopic dermatitis	Smoke
		Pollen
		Changes in weather
		Airborne chemicals or dusts
		Menstrual cycles

A diagnosis of asthma should be considered if any of these symptoms and physical examination findings is present, and if these findings are modified by the factors listed. The likelihood of asthma is increased if multiple key indicators are present. Spirometry is necessary for the actual diagnosis of asthma.

Adapted from National Heart, Lung, and Blood Institute. NIH expert panel report 3: guidelines for the diagnosis and management of asthma. 2007. Available at: http://www.nhlbi.nih.gov/guidelines/asthma/asthgdln.pdf. Accessed September 10, 2013.

days missed, ability to engage in normal daily activities, and quality of life assessments.[3] The frequency of exacerbations in the population with asthma varies widely. Importantly, the severity of disease (as measured by frequency of nighttime awakenings, usage of short-acting β_2-agonists, and interference with normal activity) does not correlate with the intensity of exacerbations.[3] Indeed, severe, life-threatening exacerbations can occur even in people with intermittent or mild asthma when provoked by an exposure, such as a viral illness, irritant, or allergen.[3] However, decreased FEV_1 in children demonstrates a strong association with the risk of asthma exacerbations.[4] In terms of modifying factors, viral infections are the most common cause of asthma exacerbations.[3]

There is a traditional division between allergic and nonallergic asthma. Allergic asthma is the subtype that accounts for approximately 50% to 80% of asthma cases, and is defined as asthma and positivity to skin prick test or specific IgE.[5,6] Allergic asthma is more common in younger males and associated with milder disease, whereas nonallergic asthma is more common in older females and more severe disease.[7,8] Nonallergic asthma exacerbations are more commonly triggered by infection, irritants, gastroesophageal reflux disease, stress, and exercise.[7] Despite the many overlapping phenotypes of asthma, the pattern of airway inflammation, the cellular profile, and the response of structural cells is consistent across all types of asthma.[3]

The asthma phenotype can be quite variable because of complex interactions between the environment and underlying genetic factors. Although asthma symptoms are typically episodic and reversible (either spontaneously or with treatment), there are also more long-term changes to the asthmatic airway that can occur from inflammation.[9] Multiple inflammatory cells and cytokines have been described in asthma pathogenesis, yet the mechanisms leading to the variability of disease phenotypes are still only partially understood.[3]

The Unified Airway, Asthma, and the Otolaryngologist

The unified airway model suggests that inflammatory diseases of the upper and lower airways are interconnected because of shared epithelial lining and inflammatory mediators. Pseudostratified columnar epithelium is the mucosal lining in the middle ear, nasal cavity, sinuses, and the lower airway, and the inflammatory mediators in chronic disease of the upper and lower airways, such as rhinosinusitis and asthma, are frequently the same (interleukin [IL]-4, IL-5, and IL-13).[10] Rhinitis, sinusitis, and asthma are frequently comorbid conditions. Indeed, a coincidence of upper and lower airway pathologies is suggested by self-reported symptoms in people with asthma, who list allergic rhinitis and sinusitis as their most common comorbidities.[11] A study by Corren[12] demonstrated the presence of rhinitis in 78% of people with asthma, and the presence of asthma in 38% of patients with rhinitis. Other conditions that otolaryngology patients frequently present with include vocal cord dysfunction, obstructive sleep apnea, and gastroesophageal reflux disease, all of which can masquerade as asthma, and can coexist with it. It is therefore important for otolaryngologists to be aware of the diagnosis and management of this common, complex, and treatable disease.

PATHOPHYSIOLOGY
Inflammation and Airway Remodeling

The inflammation in asthma is mediated by multiple cell types including mast cells, eosinophils, T lymphocytes, macrophages, neutrophils, and epithelial cells.[3] Asthma has allergic and nonallergic presentations, based on the presence or absence of IgE antibodies to common environmental allergens. Both variants are characterized by airway infiltration by T-helper (Th) cells, which secrete a predominantly Th2 milieu (cytokines IL-4, IL-5, and IL-13).[3,5] These cytokines stimulate mast cells, cause eosinophilia, promote leukocytosis, and enhance B-cell IgE production.

Although mild asthma symptoms are episodic and reversible, with disease progression and severity long-term and permanent airway changes can be present. Long-term changes can include airway smooth muscle hypertrophy and hyperplasia; increased mucus production (and associated risk of mucus plugs); and edema.[3] In the subepithelial layer, thickening can range from 7 to 23 μm, versus 4 to 5 μm in normal subjects, and more commonly affects the smaller airways (2–6 mm).[5,13,14] Permanent changes can include thickening of subbasement membrane, subepithelial edema and fibrosis, airway smooth muscle hypertrophy and hyperplasia, blood vessel proliferation and dilation, and mucus gland hyperplasia and hypersecretion.[3,14,15] Transforming growth factor-β, IL-11, and IL-17 are profibrotic factors that are increased in asthma and that lead to increased levels of types I and III collagen, resulting in subepithelial fibrosis.[16] Interestingly, most of the histopathologic findings noted previously are shared between asthma and chronic rhinosinusitis, and are worse when a patient has both conditions as opposed to either one.[15,17]

There is likely an occult process of bronchial inflammation that precedes clinical symptoms of asthma. Bronchial biopsies of children with early respiratory symptoms who progressed to asthma had higher concentrations of eosinophils in the bronchial mucosa and thicker subepithelial lamina reticularis than those who did not, and these findings were present before the clinical presentation of disease.[18] This suggests that an inflammatory milieu may precede clinical symptoms in people with asthma. Furthermore, in patients who had clinical symptoms of asthma that then seemed to go into remission, evidence of inflammation and remodeling persist on follow-up biopsies.[19–21] Clinical symptoms are a late manifestation of lower airway inflammation. Despite there being a robust response to anti-inflammatory medications with symptom control in many people with asthma, symptoms tend to recur when these drugs are no longer being used. Moreover, as in chronic rhinosinusitis, corticosteroids can result in symptom control, but they do not significantly impact the long-term inflammation in the disease process.[16] There are many treatments for asthma symptoms, but asthma is not a curable disease, and there is evidence that inflammation is life-long and occurs even when no symptoms are present.

Bronchoconstriction and Airway Hyperresponsiveness

The bronchoconstriction that occurs in asthma exacerbations is the main cause of obstructive symptoms. Airway hyperresponsiveness, or twitchy airways, occurs secondary to inflammation and airway remodeling. There is a distinct correlation between airway hyperresponsiveness and the degree of inflammation present. Bronchoconstriction can be induced by several pathways. Allergen-induced bronchoconstriction is caused by IgE-dependent mast cell degranulation, with resultant release of histamine, tryptase, leukotrienes, and prostaglandins.[22] Nonsteroidal anti-inflammatory disease–induced bronchoconstriction by the cyclooxygenase-2 pathway can also occur in susceptible patient populations.[23] (Approximately 10% of people with asthma are aspirin-sensitive.[24]) In addition to these mechanisms, bronchoconstriction by mast cell degranulation can also occur secondary to osmotic stimuli, which is likely the cause of exercise-induced bronchoconstriction.[3]

Genetics of Asthma

The genetics of asthma are complex and there are multiple genes that are thought to play a role, although there is not one specific gene that can explain most asthma cases. One landmark review article[25] stated that asthma susceptibility genes fall into four main groups: (1) genes associated with innate immunity and immunoregulation; (2) genes associated with Th2 cell differentiation and effector functions; (3) genes associated with epithelial biology and mucosal immunity; and (4) genes associated with lung function, airway remodeling, and disease severity. One study highlighted 43 replicated genes identified in the pathogenesis of asthma from well-conducted association studies, but how these genes interact with each other and the environment, and the role of epistasis in gene expression, requires further research.[26] An abundance of data demonstrates that the same polymorphism can lead to asthma pathology in one environment but not another.[25] Indeed, there is striking evidence among people with similar genetic backgrounds that environmental exposures can have a profound impact on asthma and wheezing incidence. For example, a comparison of people of Chinese origin showed a significantly increased prevalence of asthma in those living in Canada and Hong Kong versus mainland China.[27] A study of West Germany and East Germany shortly after reunification demonstrated an increased prevalence of asthma in the former.[28]

Risk Factors for Asthma

Numerous potential risk factors have been studied in relation to the development of asthma. Atopy is frequently identified as a strong risk factor for the development of asthma, yet there is not always a direct correlation between the two.[3,29] Some studies have demonstrated that early dust mite sensitization and maternal asthma are very significant predictors of asthma.[30,31] Parental smoking is a significant risk factor for acute lower respiratory tract infections in infants, and the development of wheezing and asthma in children.[32] However, there is also a high incidence of asthma in children not exposed to tobacco smoke. Active smoking in adults is associated with the development of asthma later in life.[33] Air pollution and viral infections are well-established triggers for asthma exacerbations,[34,35] but there is conflicting data as to whether these factors contribute to developing asthma.[28,36] Microbial exposure is inversely correlated with the development of asthma and atopy, and may account for the disparate prevalence of asthma in urban versus rural (specifically farming) environments.[2,37–39] Ultimately, it is likely that asthma develops in genetically susceptible individuals through a combination of complex environmental exposures.

DEMOGRAPHICS AND EPIDEMIOLOGY
Prevalence Internationally

There is wide variability in terms of the international prevalence of asthma, and methods by which international asthma prevalence is ascertained. Large, multinational studies that have attempted to characterize the epidemiology of asthma have determined its prevalence by such questions as: "Have you (has your child) had wheezing or whistling in the chest in the past 12 months?"[40] The European Community Respiratory Health Survey, a large, 22-country study, was based on an interviewer-led questionnaire and, when possible, objective measures, such as spirometry and skin prick testing.[41] Using these methods, there is a lower incidence of asthma in Asia and India (2%–4%) than in such countries as Canada, the United Kingdom, Australia, and New Zealand (15%–20%).[42] The European Community Respiratory Health Survey study showed a higher prevalence in Western Europe and the United States than in Eastern Europe.[41] Although asthma symptoms and prevalence increased in many countries from the 1960s through the 1990s, since that time there has been greater variability. In some countries asthma prevalence has increased significantly, whereas in others it has remained stable or even declined (**Fig. 1**).[2]

Prevalence in the United States

Within the United States, the overall prevalence of asthma has increased in recent years, although there is also wide variability geographically (**Fig. 2**). In 2011, asthma prevalence ranged from 5.5% in Tennessee to 18% in the District of Columbia.[43] In 2001, 7% of the overall US population (~20 million people) had asthma, whereas in 2009, 8% of the population (~25 million people) had asthma.[44] Women are more likely than men, and boys are more likely than girls to have asthma.[41,44] It is most common among African American children, who have an approximately one in six chance of having asthma, and as a group had the highest increase in asthma prevalence from 2001 to 2009.[44] People with asthma are more likely to be younger and unmarried, have lower educational attainment, be impoverished, and have comorbidities.[45] Asthma is the third leading cause of hospitalization among children younger than age 15.[46] In 2009, deaths caused by asthma totaled 3388, of which 157 were children.[47]

Costs

Asthma is associated with significant quality of life disruption, a decrease in work productivity, missed school, and increased health care costs. Multiple methods have been used to assess the overall costs of asthma, but one of the best studies was conducted by the Centers for Disease Control and Prevention, published in 2011, looking at direct medical costs and productivity losses caused by morbidity and mortality from asthma from 2002 to 2007.[45] The Centers for Disease Control and Prevention data came from the Medical Expenditure Panel Survey, a large, nationally representative survey that examined demographic and socioeconomic characteristics, employment, days disrupted by injury or illness, health care and medication use, medical conditions, and

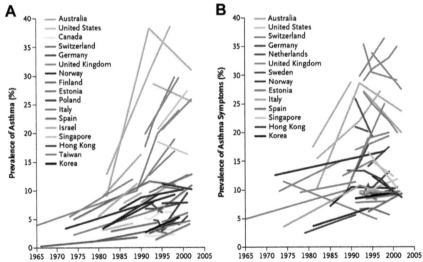

Fig. 1. Prevalence rates of asthma and asthma symptoms from around the world. Although many countries have shown increased prevalence of asthma and asthma symptoms, other countries have remained stable or even declined. (*From* Eder W, Ege MJ, von Mutius E. The asthma epidemic. N Engl J Med 2006;355:2226–35; with permission.)

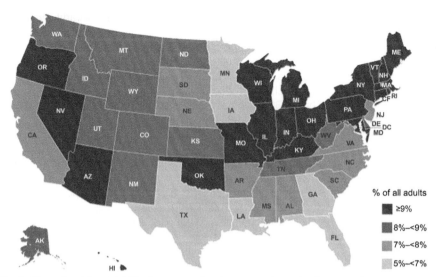

Fig. 2. There is wide variability in terms of asthma prevalence in the United States, ranging from 5.5% in Tennessee to 18% in the District of Columbia. (*From* Centers for Disease Control and Prevention. CDC vital signs. 2013. Available at: http://www.cdc.gov/VitalSigns/Asthma/index.html. Accessed September 10, 2013.)

health status. Over the 6-year period studied, costs were reported in 2009 dollars (Consumer Price Index-adjusted), as follows: the total cost per person with asthma was estimated at $3259 per year during the years 2002 to 2007. The predicted incremental cost for hospital outpatient visits was $151, for emergency department visits $110, and for inpatient visits $446.[45] On an annual basis, the cost of office-based visits for persons with asthma was estimated at $581 per year, and the additional cost of prescription medication expenditures was approximately $1680. Prescription medications accounted for the largest percentage of total medical expenditures in the adult population. This was a changing feature of asthma costs, because hospital costs accounted for most direct costs of asthma in the 1990s. Nationally, the United States population missed approximately 14.41 million work days and 3.68 million school days, with a combined estimated value of $2.03 billion per year. Overall, the study estimated that the total cost of asthma to society in 2007, including incremental direct costs and estimates of lost productivity, was approximately $56 billion.[45]

SUMMARY

Asthma is a complex disorder, affected by genetics and the environment, with a multifactorial cause and an as yet only partially understood pathophysiology. With its unifying symptoms of shortness of breath, cough, chest tightness, and/or wheezing, and its characteristic airway edema, inflammation, remodeling, and hyperresponsiveness, it is increasingly being perceived as a syndrome rather than one specific disease entity. The societal burden of asthma is substantial, and its costs and prevalence continue to increase in the United States.

REFERENCES

1. Osler W. The principles and practice of medicine. New York, London: D. Appleton and Company; 1920.

2. Eder W, Ege MJ, von Mutius E. The asthma epidemic. N Engl J Med 2006;355: 2226–35.
3. Busse WW, et al. Expert Panel Report Three. Guidelines for the diagnosis and management of asthma. National Institutes of Health; 2007.
4. Fuhlbrigge AL, Kitch BT, Paltiel AD, et al. FEV(1) is associated with risk of asthma attacks in a pediatric population. J Allergy Clin Immunol 2001;107:61–7.
5. Cohn L, Elias JA, Chupp GL. Asthma: mechanisms of disease persistence and progression. Annu Rev Immunol 2004;22:789–815.
6. Handoyo S, Rosenwasser LJ. Asthma phenotypes. Curr Allergy Asthma Rep 2009;9:439–45.
7. Novak N, Bieber T. Allergic and nonallergic forms of atopic diseases. J Allergy Clin Immunol 2003;112:252–62.
8. Romanet-Manent S, Charpin D, Magnan A, et al. Allergic vs nonallergic asthma: what makes the difference? Allergy 2002;57:607–13.
9. Holgate ST, Polosa R. The mechanisms, diagnosis, and management of severe asthma in adults. Lancet 2006;368:780–93.
10. Bachert C, Vignola AM, Gevaert P, et al. Allergic rhinitis, rhinosinusitis, and asthma: one airway disease. Immunol Allergy Clin North Am 2004;24:19–43.
11. Dixon AE, Kaminsky DA, Holbrook JT, et al. Allergic rhinitis and sinusitis in asthma: differential effects on symptoms and pulmonary function. Chest 2006; 130:429–35.
12. Corren J. Allergic rhinitis and asthma: how important is the link? J Allergy Clin Immunol 1997;99:S781–6.
13. Roberts CR, Okazawa M, Wiggs B, et al. Airway wall thickening. In: Barnes PJ, Grunstein MM, Leff AR, et al, editors. Asthma. Philadelphia: Raven Publishers; 1997. p. 925–35.
14. Homer RJ, Elias JA. Consequences of long-term inflammation. Airway remodeling. Clin Chest Med 2000;21:331–43, ix.
15. Krouse JH, Brown RW, Fineman SM, et al. Asthma and the unified airway. Otolaryngol Head Neck Surg 2007;136:S75–106.
16. Chakir J, Shannon J, Molet S, et al. Airway remodeling-associated mediators in moderate to severe asthma: effect of steroids on TGF-beta, IL-11, IL-17, and type I and type III collagen expression. J Allergy Clin Immunol 2003;111:1293–8.
17. Dhong HJ, Kim HY, Cho DY. Histopathologic characteristics of chronic sinusitis with bronchial asthma. Acta Otolaryngol 2005;125:169–76.
18. Pohunek P, Warner JO, Turzíková J, et al. Markers of eosinophilic inflammation and tissue re-modelling in children before clinically diagnosed bronchial asthma. Pediatr Allergy Immunol 2005;16:43–51.
19. van Den Toorn LM, Prins JB, Overbeek SE, et al. Adolescents in clinical remission of atopic asthma have elevated exhaled nitric oxide levels and bronchial hyperresponsiveness. Am J Respir Crit Care Med 2000;162:953–7.
20. van den Toorn LM, Overbeek SE, de Jongste JC, et al. Airway inflammation is present during clinical remission of atopic asthma. Am J Respir Crit Care Med 2001; 164:2107–13.
21. van den Toorn LM, Overbeek SE, Prins JB, et al. Asthma remission: does it exist? Curr Opin Pulm Med 2003;9:15–20.
22. Busse WW, Lemanske RF. Asthma. N Engl J Med 2001;344:350–62.
23. Stevenson DD, Szczeklik A. Clinical and pathologic perspectives on aspirin sensitivity and asthma. J Allergy Clin Immunol 2006;118:773–86 [quiz: 787–8].
24. Vally H, Taylor ML, Thompson PJ. The prevalence of aspirin intolerant asthma (AIA) in Australian asthmatic patients. Thorax 2002;57:569–74.

25. Vercelli D. Discovering susceptibility genes for asthma and allergy. Nat Rev Immunol 2008;8:169–82.
26. Weiss ST, Raby BA, Rogers A. Asthma genetics and genomics 2009. Curr Opin Genet Dev 2009;19:279–82.
27. Wang HY, Wong GW, Chen YZ, et al. Prevalence of asthma among Chinese adolescents living in Canada and in China. CMAJ 2008;179:1133–42.
28. von Mutius E, Martinez FD, Fritzsch C, et al. Prevalence of asthma and atopy in two areas of West and East Germany. Am J Respir Crit Care Med 1994;149: 358–64.
29. Priftanji A, Strachan D, Burr M, et al. Asthma and allergy in Albania and the UK. Lancet 2001;358:1426–7.
30. Lau S, Illi S, Sommerfeld C, et al. Early exposure to house-dust mite and cat allergens and development of childhood asthma: a cohort study. Multicentre Allergy Study Group. Lancet 2000;356:1392–7.
31. Sears MR, Herbison GP, Holdaway MD, et al. The relative risks of sensitivity to grass pollen, house dust mite and cat dander in the development of childhood asthma. Clin Exp Allergy 1989;19:419–24.
32. Strachan DP, Cook DG. Health effects of passive smoking. 6. Parental smoking and childhood asthma: longitudinal and case-control studies. Thorax 1998;53: 204–12.
33. Strachan DP, Butland BK, Anderson HR. Incidence and prognosis of asthma and wheezing illness from early childhood to age 33 in a national British cohort. BMJ 1996;312:1195–9.
34. Patel MM, Miller RL. Air pollution and childhood asthma: recent advances and future directions. Curr Opin Pediatr 2009;21:235–42.
35. Corne JM, Marshall C, Smith S, et al. Frequency, severity, and duration of rhinovirus infections in asthmatic and non-asthmatic individuals: a longitudinal cohort study. Lancet 2002;359:831–4.
36. von Mutius E. Infection: friend or foe in the development of atopy and asthma? The epidemiological evidence. Eur Respir J 2001;18:872–81.
37. Braun-Fahrländer C, Lauener R. Farming and protective agents against allergy and asthma. Clin Exp Allergy 2003;33:409–11.
38. Keeley DJ, Neill P, Gallivan S. Comparison of the prevalence of reversible airways obstruction in rural and urban Zimbabwean children. Thorax 1991;46:549–53.
39. van Strien RT, Engel R, Holst O, et al. Microbial exposure of rural school children, as assessed by levels of N-acetyl-muramic acid in mattress dust, and its association with respiratory health. J Allergy Clin Immunol 2004;113:860–7.
40. Asher MI, Montefort S, Björkstén B, et al. Worldwide time trends in the prevalence of symptoms of asthma, allergic rhinoconjunctivitis, and eczema in childhood: ISAAC Phases One and Three repeat multicountry cross-sectional surveys. Lancet 2006;368:733–43.
41. Janson C, Anto J, Burney P, et al. The European Community Respiratory Health Survey: what are the main results so far? European Community Respiratory Health Survey II. Eur Respir J 2001;18:598–611.
42. Subbarao P, Mandhane PJ, Sears MR. Asthma: epidemiology, etiology and risk factors. CMAJ 2009;181:E181–90.
43. Centers for Disease Control and Prevention. Behavioral risk factor surveillance survey. Available at: http://www.lung.org/lung-disease/asthma/resources/facts-and-figures/asthma-children-fact-sheet.html. Accessed July 4, 2013.
44. Centers for Disease Control and Prevention. CDC vital signs. 2013. Available at: http://www.cdc.gov/VitalSigns/Asthma/index.html. Accessed July 4, 2013.

45. Barnett SB, Nurmagambetov TA. Costs of asthma in the United States: 2002-2007. J Allergy Clin Immunol 2011;127:145–52.
46. Centers for Disease Control and Prevention. National Center for Health Statistics, National Hospital Discharge Survey, 1995-2010. 2013. Available at: http://www.lung.org/lung-disease/asthma/resources/facts-and-figures/asthma-children-fact-sheet.html. Accessed July 4, 2013.
47. Centers for Disease Control and Prevention. Statistics. Compiled from Compressed Mortality File 1999-2009 Series 1920 No. 1920.

Asthma: Symptoms and Presentation

Monica Oberoi Patadia, MD[a], Lauren L. Murrill, MD[a],
Jacquelynne Corey, MD[b],*

KEYWORDS

- Asthma symptoms ● Asthma presentation ● Wheezing ● Cough ● Pediatric asthma
- Asthma differential diagnosis

KEY POINTS

- The four main symptoms of asthma are wheezing, cough, chest tightness, and dyspnea.
- A thorough history taking is essential—personal, family, and social histories must be obtained.
- Infants and preschoolers must be diagnosed based on presentation, history, and physical examination because objective measures cannot easily be used.
- Asthma in the elderly is underdiagnosed and often compounded by comorbidities.
- The physical examination can help distinguish the severity of the asthma exacerbation.

OVERVIEW

Asthma is a common diagnosis in both outpatient and emergency department settings. It has a varied presentation between patients and between each exacerbation. Hence, understanding the common symptoms and presentations is essential to correctly diagnosing this disease.

This article discusses the symptoms of asthma, age-related key points, variables and differential diagnoses, the classification of acute asthma attacks, physical examination essentials, and risk factors for development and death from this disease process.

SYMPTOMS

Asthma is defined as a reversible airway obstruction that presents with some combination of wheezing, dyspnea, airway hyperresponsiveness, cough, and mucus hypersecretion.[1] The 4 most common presenting symptoms are wheezing, cough,

[a] Department of Otolaryngology – Head and Neck Surgery, Loyola University Medical Center, 2160 South First Avenue, Building 105, Room 1870, Maywood, IL 60153, USA; [b] Section of Otolaryngology – Head and Neck Surgery, Department of Surgery, University of Chicago, 5841 South Maryland Avenue, MC 1035, Chicago, IL 60637, USA
* Corresponding author.
E-mail address: jcorey@surgery.bsd.uchicago.edu

Otolaryngol Clin N Am 47 (2014) 23–32
http://dx.doi.org/10.1016/j.otc.2013.10.001
0030-6665/14/$ – see front matter © 2014 Elsevier Inc. All rights reserved.

shortness of breath, and a subjective sensation of chest tightness.[2] Although asthma can have a variable presentation, this is the main constellation of symptoms. One or more of these symptoms are present during an asthma attack. Not only does the presentation vary between people but also a single patient may have extreme variation between each exacerbation.

Asthma is often described as a chronic disease with intermittent symptoms and acute exacerbations. It is reported, however, that up to 27% of people with asthma have daily symptoms.[3] Although asthma can occur in any age group, in Western countries it is known as the most common chronic disease of childhood.[4] Classically, younger patients present with recurrent wheezing and/or coughing episodes that may or may not be accompanied by chest tightness or dyspnea[3]; 80% of patients have a slow onset of asthma symptoms with progressive deterioration over a period of 6 or more hours.[5]

Because this presentation has a broad differential diagnosis, patients' exposure to allergens or triggers and their response to bronchodilators are of key importance. These topics are discussed further by Ferguson and colleagues elsewhere in this issue. See **Table 1** for a concise summary.

Wheezing

Wheezing, most commonly on expiration, is the hallmark symptom of an acute asthma exacerbation. Wheezing is neither sensitive nor specific, however, and the presence of wheezing is not necessary in order to diagnose asthma. Additionally, there are multiple other disease processes that may present with wheezing.

Wheezing is defined as a musical, high-pitched, whistling sound produced by airflow turbulence. The sound occurs due to airflow passing through narrowed bronchioles.[1,6] Wheezing may not carry an obvious pattern during the respiratory cycle but rather is noted at various, seemingly random, points during respiration. Wheezing varies in tone and duration over time. The characteristics of the wheeze often clue a physician to the degree of exacerbation. A mild exacerbation presents with only end-expiratory wheezing. A severe exacerbation usually has both inspiratory and expiratory wheezing present. In its most severe form, patients may have an absence, or loss, of wheezing, which denotes a significantly narrowed airway with limited airflow. This is indicative of impending respiratory failure and respiratory muscle fatigue.[7]

Should a patient present with wheezing, it is essential to consider diagnoses other than asthma by combining symptoms, physical examination, and diagnostic testing, such as spirometry, methacholine challenge, and/or a bronchodilator trial. Chapter 5 discusses diagnostic testing in further details. If wheezing clears with cough, for example, a secretion issue may be suspected. If a wheeze is monophasic and begins

Table 1 Asthma: common symptoms and physical examination findings	
Common symptoms	• Wheezing • Cough • Chest tightness • Dyspnea
Common physical examination findings	• Breathlessness • Tachycardia • Audible wheezing • Atopic findings, such as rhinitis and eczema

and ends consistently at the same point of each respiratory cycle, local bronchial narrowing due to foreign body or bronchogenic carcinoma should be considered.

Cough and Mucus Production

Cough is another common presenting symptom of asthma. Many patients emphasize that their cough is present nocturnally, especially from midnight until the early morning hours, and describe it as nonproductive.[7] If sputum is present, it is usually clear mucoid or pale yellow in appearance. In the pediatric population, the frequency of coughing is thought related to the amount of neutrophils present in the sputum, suggesting an infectious cause in this group of patients. Because cough is occasionally the only symptom, chronic cough in adults should prompt a work-up for asthma, especially if symptoms are seasonal or if the cough presents after trigger exposure.[1,8] At times, cough is the only symptom and is described in the literature as cough-variant asthma or cough-equivalent asthma; this form is rarely accompanied by wheezing or dyspnea.[1] There is also exercise-induced asthma, which often presents with cough. These specific forms of asthma are discussed by Ryan and colleagues elsewhere in this issue.

Although discussed less in the literature, the presence of increased mucus production can also indicate asthma when combined with other symptoms. Up to 9% of patients have profuse sputum production during attacks due to impairment of mucociliary clearance. When present, this often signifies poor asthma control.[1]

Chest Tightness

A subjective symptom that is commonly described is chest tightness. Although this can be present in any form of asthma, it is often seen in exercise-induced and nocturnal asthma. Often it is referred to as a generalized chest pain, a sensation of chest congestion, or difficulty with deep inspiration. Patients describe it as a band-like constriction or a heavy weight, rarely a sharp pain. This, too, may be the only symptom or may be part of a constellation of symptoms. Unfortunately, this complaint is not specific and is seen in multiple cardiac, pulmonary, and gastrointestinal conditions. Therefore, an isolated symptom of chest tightness must be thoroughly worked up for other serious and life-threatening conditions prior to arriving at the conclusion of asthma.

Dyspnea

Dyspnea is a subjective sensation of shortness of breath. Often patients describe this as "difficulty breathing." Again, dyspnea does not imply asthma and must be evaluated in a larger context.

History Taking

Given the nonspecific signs of asthma (discussed previously), it is essential to take a thorough history when patients present with symptoms. The discussion should focus on personal, family, and social histories. Clinical symptoms should be described by the patient or parent in terms of intensity, duration, frequency, environmental exposure, nocturnal frequency, and seasonal components.[9] A patient's personal history is of utmost importance. Indicators in a patient's history that make asthma more likely include a history of atopy or dry cough.[3,10–12] Allergy is a trigger in 60% to 90% of children and in half of adults.[12] The physician should elucidate a patient's exacerbation history—What are the usual prodromal signs and symptoms? How quickly did this attack come on? Are there any associated illnesses or comorbidities? How many attacks, emergency room visits, and hospitalizations have there been in the past year? Has an attack ever required intubation?

Many patients describe a personal or family history that includes asthma, allergies, sinusitis, rhinitis, and/or eczema, indicating a genetic predisposition to atopy and likely atopic component to the asthma diagnosis. Nasal polyps and/or a history of aspirin sensitivity may occur with asthma. This is also known as aspirin-exacerbated respiratory disease (AERD). Social history is important to determine a patient's contact with possible triggers, whether environmental, such as tobacco exposure, or work related. Elsewhere in this issue, Ferguson and his colleagues discusses asthma triggers in greater detail.

ASTHMA BY AGE GROUP
Infants/Preschoolers

Infants and preschoolers are particularly challenging to evaluate and work-up because they are unable to participate in subjective questioning or diagnostic studies. Despite this, preschool age is commonly the first time that patients have their first asthma attack.[6] The diagnosis must be made on symptoms, physical examination, risk factors, and response to treatment because objective measures cannot be used. The pattern of their disease usually includes brief, recurrent exacerbations of coughing and wheezing.[13] On presentation, this age group usually has cough, wheezing, and prolonged expiration. In addition, they frequently feel anxious.[4] Older children often complain of chest tightness or recurrent chest congestion.[7]

There are a few additional presentations that should clue physicians to the possibility of an asthma diagnosis in this age group. The children often have nonspecific symptoms that are diagnosed as other diseases, such as recurrent bronchitis or bronchiolitis, recurrent pneumonia, or croup. Parents often describe persistent cough associated with colds and viruses. Most children who have chronic or recurrent bronchitis or pneumonia have asthma as an underlying diagnosis.[7] In school-aged children, asthma exacerbations peak in early September and are least common in the summer months.

It is thought that in young children, up to 85% of wheezing episodes are triggered by viral infections, suggesting causation for the overlap of the disease entities discussed previously. Most commonly, respiratory syncytial virus and rhinovirus are implicated as viral triggers. A strong association was found between rhinovirus-associated wheezing requiring hospitalization during the first 2 years of life and childhood asthma. The risk of developing childhood asthma in this population was 4-fold the risk compared with children presenting with other viral illnesses.[14–16] Unlike older children and adolescents, preschoolers have less impairment from their disease process.[13]

The probability of asthma as the primary diagnosis in pediatric patients increases if they present with more than 1 of the 4 common symptoms of asthma. From the history, it should be gathered whether the current symptoms are separate from a recent cold or infection, if the symptoms are frequent or recurrent, if they are worse at night or in the early morning, and if they are associated with exercise or known triggers. Parents may describe severe episodes of wheezing or dyspnea that began after 1 year of age and/or a chronic cough. All of these make the diagnosis of asthma more probable.[10,17] Common comorbidities in pediatric patients with asthma include gastroesophageal reflux disease (GERD), rhinosinusitis, dysfunctional breathing, obesity, and food allergy.[18–20] Asthma symptoms in the face of any of these diagnoses should trigger a suspicion for asthma.

There are 3 wheezing phenotypes that have been described in the preschool-aged population. These have been used to help determine if asthma will be present later in life. The early transient phenotype begins in the first 3 years of life and resolves by age 6. Persistent wheezers also initiate wheezing episodes before age 3, but these continue to persist at age 6. Late-onset wheezing does not begin until a patient is between 3 and 6 years old. Transient early wheezers often outgrow their symptoms. Those with persistent or late-onset wheezing are more likely to have symptoms into adolescence and adulthood.[10,13] If recurrent wheezing is present in the first 3 years of life, a child is at a 4.7 times greater risk of developing asthma. If the wheezing persists or is present in years 4 through 6, the risk is 15 times that of the general population.[1]

Elderly

Asthma in the elderly is more common than many physicians realize, and being aware of the possibility in this age group is essential to providing appropriate care. Whereas asthma is frequently diagnosed in childhood, it is often underdiagnosed and undertreated in the elderly (age >65) population. After the age group birth to 4 years old, patients over 65 have the highest rate of office or emergency department visits for asthma. Difficulties of diagnosis in this age group are not only their physiologic age-related changes in respiratory and immune status but also their decreased awareness of subjective symptoms, such as dyspnea, making a delay in diagnosis common.[21] Symptoms are the same as in younger patients, but the differential diagnosis is much broader for an elderly population (discussed later). Additionally, asthma presents in the face of other comorbidities, and the symptoms associated with asthma often are swept into another diagnosis.[22] Another difficult differentiation lies between asthma and chronic obstructive pulmonary disease (COPD). There are many patients with both diagnoses and asthma activity is increased in patients with COPD.[23] The preferred way to differentiate between an asthma and COPD exacerbation is not symptoms or presentation but via diagnostic testing.[21] See **Table 2** for a concise summary.

DIFFERENTIAL DIAGNOSES

The differential diagnosis of patients presenting with symptoms of asthma is broad and can be best broken down by age group.

Neonates and Children

In the neonatal and pediatric population, cystic fibrosis and congenital anomalies, such as a vascular ring, primary ciliary dyskinesia, esophageal fistula, foreign body, bronchiolitis, cardiac disease, and bronchomalacia or tracheomalacia, may present with symptoms mimicking asthma and should be ruled out. Signs that may point a practitioner to a direction other than asthma in the young population include symptoms presenting at or shortly after birth, continuous wheezing, failure to thrive, failure to respond to medications, and lack of an association with usual triggers.[13]

Table 2 Differential diagnoses by age group	
Neonates and children	Cystic fibrosis, congenital abnormalities, primary ciliary dyskinesia, esophageal fistula, foreign body ingestion, bronchiolitis, cardiac disease, bronchomalacia or tracheomalacia
Adults	COPD, congestive heart failure, valvular heart disease, pneumonia, chronic aspiration, allergic bronchopulmonary aspergillosis, laryngeal edema, neoplasm, foreign body ingestion, vocal cord dysfunction, pulmonary embolism, noncardiogenic pulmonary edema, GERD

Adults

In adults, multiple disease processes can present with wheezing, cough, dyspnea, or chest tightness. In those presenting with dyspnea, the most common diagnosis is not asthma but rather cardiac or other pulmonary disorders, such as COPD.[21] Cardiac causes, such as congestive heart failure or valvular heart disease, should be considered. Other respiratory entities, such as COPD, pneumonia, chronic aspiration, and allergic bronchpulmonary aspergillosis, may present this way. Airway obstruction or abnormalities in the form of laryngeal edema, neoplasm, foreign body, or vocal cord dysfunction may mimic asthma symptoms. Less commonly, endobronchial disease, tracheobronchial stenosis, pulmonary embolism, and noncardiogenic pulmonary edema should be on the differential. Commonly, GERD may mimic asthma in presentation and is often a comorbidity, clouding the acute presentation and work-up.

CLASSIFICATION OF ACUTE ASTHMA EXACERBATIONS

There are 4 general classifications of acute asthma exacerbations that are described in the literature and used to direct diagnosis and management.

Mild

Patients presenting with mild attacks usually are breathless after physical activity and are able to talk in complete sentences. At rest, they may have minimal symptoms. They are usually not agitated. On examination, they are able to lie flat without becoming dyspneic. They often have an elevated respiratory rate but are not using accessory muscles. They have a heart rate of less than 100 beats per minute and oxygenate well on room air. Frequently, moderate end-expiratory wheezing can be heard.

Moderately Severe

In moderately severe attacks, patients often have a hard time speaking in full sentences and become breathless when talking. Infants have recent feeding issues and a soft cry. Respiratory rate is elevated and accessory muscle use is often noted on respiration. Pediatric patients may appear in more noticeable distress with supraclavicular or intercostal retractions as well as nasal flaring and abdominal breathing. Mild tachycardia, usually less than 120 beats per minute, is seen. Loud expiratory wheezing is noted and oxygen saturations on room air start to fall into the low 90s at this stage. Additionally, pulsus paradoxus may be present. Pulsus paradoxus is defined as an abnormally large decrease in systolic blood pressure during inspiration. Normal variation is less than 10 mm Hg and when it becomes greater than this, pulsus paradoxus is said to be present.

Severe

Severe exacerbations are characterized by breathlessness at rest, an inability to eat, lie down, or talk in full sentences. Patients are often agitated and may be sitting in the tripod position: hunched over with their hands supporting their torso. In addition to tachypnea and tachycardia, oxygen saturation is usually less than 91% and supplemental oxygen is frequently required. Loud biphasic wheezing is heard and accessory muscle use with suprasternal retractions is common. Sinus tachycardia is most common, although supraventricular tachycardia can occur.[24] In most instances, pulsus paradoxus is present.

Imminent Respiratory Arrest

The most concerning of attacks is imminent respiratory arrest. Most alarming is when wheezing and pulsus paradoxus are absent because this indicates respiratory muscle fatigue. Profuse diaphoresis and patients subjectively feeling they cannot breathe are not uncommon. Pediatric patients are often drowsy and confused. Adolescents and adults are often already in respiratory failure if this stage of altered mental status is present. It is essential not to delay intubation if a patient presents with apnea or a coma. The need for intubation is highly probable if a patient is hypercapnic, is exhausted, or has a depressed mental status.[2] In contrast to the tachycardia (discussed previously), bradycardia may ensue due to severe hypoxemia. Often on examination, not only is wheezing absent but also no breath sounds can be heard on auscultation.[7] See **Table 3** for a concise summary.

PHYSICAL EXAMINATION

In asthma patients, a physical examination allows assessment of the severity of the exacerbation (discussed previously). The main focus of the physical examination should be to gain an idea of vital signs as well as mental and respiratory status. The physical examination is of utmost importance in infants or preschool-aged patients who present with asthma symptoms, because they are unable to perform objective measures to aid in diagnosis.[2]

In addition to vital signs, general appearance, and cardiovascular and pulmonary examinations, the head and neck examination and skin examination are essential to a thorough physical examination for patients suspected of having asthma. Another important point is that the physical examination can be normal in patients with asthma. When there are physical manifestations of the disease, many patients have atopic findings and evidence of rhinitis, furthering the belief that asthma is often allergic in nature.[25] It is essential to evaluate for conjunctival congestion and inflammation, ocular shiners, a transverse crease on the nose known as the allergic salute, pale violaceous nasal mucosa, and erythematous and boggy turbinates with or without polyps. If polyps are present, it is important to ask about aspirin sensitivity to determine if a

Table 3
Physical examination findings based on asthma exacerbation severity and classification

Classification	Vital Signs	General Examination	Respiratory Examination
Mild	• Elevated RR • HR <100 • O$_2$ sat >95%	• Complete sentences • ± Agitation	• Moderate end-expiratory wheezing
Moderate severe	• Elevated RR • HR 100–120 • O$_2$ sat low 90s • ± Pulsus paradoxus	• Unable to speak in full sentences	• ± Accessory muscle use • Loud expiratory wheezing
Severe	• Elevated RR • HR >120 • O$_2$ <91% • Pulsus paradoxus	• Breathless at rest • Inability to lie down • Agitated	• Loud biphasic wheezing • Accessory muscle use
Imminent respiratory failure	• Absent pulsus paradoxus • Bradycardia	• Diaphoresis • Altered mental status	• Absent wheezing • Absent breath sounds

Abbreviations: HR, heart rate; O$_2$ sat, oxygen saturation; RR, respiratory rate.

patient has AERD/Samter's triad—a constellation of asthma, chronic rhinosinusitis, and nasal polyposis—and aspirin sensitivity consistent with aspirin-induced asthma. The skin examination may show atopic dermatitis or eczema. Lichenified plaques in a flexural distribution characterize atopic dermatitis and approximately one-third of patients with atopic dermatitis develop asthma. If other findings are detected, such as finger clubbing, another diagnosis should be pursued.[7]

Repeat physical examination after bronchodilator trial is essential. If a patient is having a severe exacerbation, reassessment should be completed after the initial dose of bronchodilators. Other patients should be assessed after 3 doses or within 60 to 90 minutes of initial presentation.[2]

RISK FACTORS

Many risk factors exist for the development of asthma. Of these, obesity and atopy are commonly studied. Presence of obesity correlates with a more severe form of asthma that is usually not atopic in nature. Studies have found a complex temporal relationship between the onset of childhood obesity and the risk of asthma. It was determined that children overweight at the age of 1 have a decreased risk of asthma. Children with normal weight at age 1 but who had become obese by the age of 5, however, were at increased risk of developing asthma. There is also thought to be a positive relationship between maternal body mass index and childhood asthma risk.[26]

The presence of asthma should also be investigated in patients with atopic complaints, such as rhinitis and atopic dermatitis.[27–29] Other risk factors include smoking, air pollution, vitamin D deficiency, and poverty. Exposure to smoke, via personal smoking history or environmental exposure, is strongly correlated to childhood asthma and negatively correlated to the chance for remission of the disease.[26]

Given that asthma is a common disease, the consequences of severe, uncontrolled asthma are occasionally overlooked. Physicians must be vigilant to detect risk factors associated with death from asthma. These include a history of sudden, severe exacerbations; prior admissions to an intensive care unit; history of need for intubation; 2 or more hospitalizations or 3 or more emergency department visits in the past year; difficulty for patients to detect severity of symptoms; psychosocial issues; illicit drug use; low socioeconomic status; use of more than 2 canisters per month of inhaled short-acting β-agonist; and current use of systemic steroids or recent withdrawal from use of systemic steroids.[24]

SUMMARY

Given the frequency with which asthma is encountered in clinical settings, practitioners must be comfortable with evaluating the symptoms and presentation of this disease. In this article, an explanation of common symptoms and presentations for various age groups are discussed as well as the differential diagnoses of these nonspecific symptoms. The 4 categories of asthma exacerbations and the ways in which a physical examination can help determine into which category a patient falls are also outlined. This is helpful for determining severity and management, which are discussed in more detail by Schofield elsewhere in this issue.

REFERENCES

1. Gordon BR. Asthma history and presentation. Otolaryngol Clin North Am 2008; 41(2):375–85, vii–viii.

2. Camargo CA Jr, Rachelefsky G, Schatz M. Managing asthma exacerbations in the emergency department: summary of the national asthma education and prevention program expert panel report 3 guidelines for the management of asthma exacerbations. J Emerg Med 2009;37(Suppl 2):S6–17.

3. Yawn BP. Differential assessment and management of asthma vs chronic obstructive pulmonary disease. Medscape J Med 2009;11(1):20.

4. Oymar K, Halvorsen T. Emergency presentation and management of acute severe asthma in children. Scand J Trauma Resusc Emerg Med 2009;17:40. http://dx.doi.org/10.1186/1757-7241-17-40.

5. Nowak RM, Tokarski GF. Asthma. In: Marx JA, Hockberger RS, Walls RM, et al, editors. Rosen's emergency medicine: concepts and clinical practice. 7th edition. Philadelphia: Elsevier; 2010. Chapter 71.

6. Baena-Cagnani CE, Badellino HA. Diagnosis of allergy and asthma in childhood. Curr Allergy Asthma Rep 2011;11(1):71–7.

7. Morris MJ. Asthma clinical presentation. Medscape Reference. 2013. Available at: http://emedicine.medscape.com/article/296301-clinical. Accessed April 2, 2013.

8. Goldsobel AB, Kelkar PS. The adult with chronic cough. J Allergy Clin Immunol 2012;130(3):825–825.e6.

9. Spector SL, Nicklas RA, Berstein IL, et al. Practice parameters for the diagnosis and treatment of asthma. J Allergy Clin Immunol 1995;96:707–80.

10. Becker A, Lemiere C, Berube D, et al. Summary of recommendations from the canadian asthma consensus guidelines, 2003. CMAJ 2005;173(Suppl 6):S3–11.

11. Boulay ME, Morin A, Laprise C, et al. Asthma and rhinitis: what is the relationship? Curr Opin Allergy Clin Immunol 2012;12(5):449–54.

12. Li JT, Pearlman DS, Nicklas RA, et al. Algorithm for the diagnosis and management of asthma: a practice parameter update. Ann Allergy Asthma Immunol 1998;81:415–20.

13. Bacharier LB, Guilbert TW. Diagnosis and management of early asthma in preschool-aged children. J Allergy Clin Immunol 2012;130(2):287–96 [quiz: 297–8].

14. Caramori G, Papadopoulos N, Contoli M, et al. Asthma: a chronic infectious disease? Clin Chest Med 2012;33(3):473–84.

15. Castro-Rodriguez JA. The asthma predictive index: early diagnosis of asthma. Curr Opin Allergy Clin Immunol 2011;11(3):157–61.

16. Fanta CH. Diagnosis of asthma in adolescents and adults. In: Rose BD, editor. UpToDate. Waltham (MA): UpToDate; 2005.

17. Asthma guideline update. Paediatr Nurs 2008;20(5):29.

18. Bush A, Saglani S. Management of severe asthma in children. Lancet 2010; 376(9743):814–25.

19. Bush A, Zar HJ. WHO universal definition of severe asthma. Curr Opin Allergy Clin Immunol 2011;11(2):115–21.

20. Hedlin G, Konradsen J, Bush A. An update on paediatric asthma. Eur Respir Rev 2012;21(125):175–85.

21. Hanania NA, King MJ, Braman SS, et al. Asthma in the elderly: current understanding and future research needs–a report of a national institute on aging (NIA) workshop. J Allergy Clin Immunol 2011;128(Suppl 3):S4–24.

22. Yorganciioglu A, Sakar Coskun A. Is the diagnosis of asthma different in elderly? Tuberk Toraks 2012;60(1):81–5.

23. Apter AJ. Advances in adult asthma diagnosis and treatment in 2012: potential therapeutics and gene-environment interactions. J Allergy Clin Immunol 2013; 131(1):47–54.

24. Papiris S, Kotanidou A, Malagari K, et al. Clinical review: severe asthma. Crit Care 2002;6(1):30–44.
25. Azevedo P, Correia de Sousa J, Bousquet J, et al. Control of allergic rhinitis and asthma test (CARAT): dissemination and applications in primary care. Prim Care Respir J 2013;22(1):112–6.
26. Anto JM. Recent advances in the epidemiologic investigation of risk factors for asthma: a review of the 2011 literature. Curr Allergy Asthma Rep 2012;12(3): 192–200.
27. Bousquet J, Schunemann HJ, Samolinski B, et al. Allergic rhinitis and its impact on asthma (ARIA): achievements in 10 years and future needs. J Allergy Clin Immunol 2012;130(5):1049–62.
28. British Thoracic Society, Scottish Intercollegiate Guidelines Network. British guideline on the management of asthma. Thorax 2003;58(Suppl 1):i1–94.
29. Browne LR, Gorelick MH. Asthma and pneumonia. Pediatr Clin North Am 2010; 57(6):1347–56.

Asthma Diagnosis in Otolaryngology Practice
Pulmonary Function Testing

John H. Krouse, MD, PhD[a],*, Helene J. Krouse, PhD, APN-BC, CORLN[b]

KEYWORDS

- Spirometry • Asthma • Flow-volume loop • Pulmonary function testing
- Allergic rhinitis

KEY POINTS

- Current evidence-based guidelines strongly recommend the use of objective testing in the diagnosis and treatment of patients with asthma.
- Spirometry provides an easy, readily available, and inexpensive methodology that can be used in the otolaryngology office.
- Peak flow measurement can be used by patients at home to monitor their symptoms and disease status.

As previously discussed in this issue, the diagnosis of asthma is based on a comprehensive assessment of patient symptoms and signs from physical examination. In addition, there are several standardized instruments that can assist in clarifying the diagnosis and assessing the severity of the disease. Current National Heart, Lung and Blood Institute guidelines[1] recommend the use of these elements to confirm an initial diagnosis and evaluate response to therapy.

Although assessing clinical symptoms and signs can be useful in patient management, these factors can be less reliable and objective than desired, especially in their ability to quantify the physiologic expression of the disease. Because asthma represents a disease of airflow obstruction in the small bronchioles, an objective assessment of the degree of obstruction is useful in determining the degree of direct impact on pulmonary function and following both the progression of the disease and the response to medical intervention. To assist with physiologic measurement of lung function, several specific methods have been developed that can reliably and accurately assessment the impact of asthma on respiratory physiology.

[a] Department of Otolaryngology-Head and Neck Surgery, Temple University School of Medicine, 3440 North Broad Street, Kresge West #300, Philadelphia, PA 19140, USA; [b] College of Nursing, Wayne State University, 5557 Cass Avenue, Detroit, MI 48202, USA
* Corresponding author.
E-mail address: jkrouse@temple.edu

Otolaryngol Clin N Am 47 (2014) 33–37
http://dx.doi.org/10.1016/j.otc.2013.09.009
0030-6665/14/$ – see front matter © 2014 Elsevier Inc. All rights reserved.

PEAK FLOW MEASUREMENT

Peak flow meters are small, inexpensive devices that are simple to use and ideal for home assessment of pulmonary function. They primarily measure airflow through the larger portions of the airway, and are therefore less sensitive to small changes in the distal bronchioles. Their major value is for following lung function at home on a daily or twice daily basis to detect sequential changes over time. Although peak flow testing can be useful as a gross assessment of function, results are dependent on patient effort so education on proper technique is essential to obtain accurate results. In addition, beneficial use requires consistent measurement and recording on a regular basis, with poor patient or parent adherence compromising maximal benefit.

PULMONARY FUNCTION TESTING

The primary method used to assess respiratory physiology and status in patients diagnosed with or suspected of having asthma is pulmonary function testing (PFT). PFTs represent an integral portion of the diagnosis and therapeutic management of patients with asthma, and serve 3 core functions in practice: (1) to assess the presence and severity of asthma; (2) to establish reversibility of airway obstruction; and (3) to measure response to therapy. PFTs play an essential role in the management of patients suspected of having respiratory dysfunction, and can be considered an objective assessment of lung function much as audiometry represents an objective assessment of auditory function.

PFTs are important in differentiating specific pulmonary pathophysiology based on whether the disease is obstructive or restrictive, and whether obstruction is reversible or irreversible. PFTs also establish a reliable and valid baseline for establishing an initial diagnosis and for monitoring changes over time, with or without specific treatment. Because of advancements in measurement and computing technology, small, portable, inexpensive, and automated devices are now widely available for in-office use.

Physiologic testing of lung function involves several specific testing methodologies to assess components of normal pulmonary physiology, including mechanics of the lungs and ventilatory function, the ventilation-perfusion relationship, diffusion and gas exchange, and muscular strength. Full battery PFTs can include a variety of these procedures, although in the diagnosis of asthma not all components of the testing battery are necessary. The 4 primary procedures in common use include: (1) measurement of lung volume; (2) measurement of diffusing capacity; (3) spirometry; and (4) bronchoprovocation. The first of these 2 procedures is briefly reviewed here; spirometry and bronchoprovocation are discussed in greater detail.

Spirometry

Spirometry is the most commonly performed lung function study, and is often sufficient to confirm a diagnosis of asthma without more specialized testing. It can be easily and quickly performed in the office setting under the guidance and supervision of a trained technician or health care provider. Spirometry measures air flow in the lungs, which involves assessing how much air can move in and out of the lungs as well as how fast the air in the lungs can be exhaled. The indications for spirometry include the diagnosis and monitoring of suspected diseases of lung function, including asthma, chronic obstructive pulmonary disease, and other common and uncommon pulmonary conditions.

Spirometry involves a maneuver in which the patient voluntarily inhales maximally and then rapidly and forcefully exhales to the fullest extent possible. At full inspiration, the patient has filled the lungs with air, and at full expiration some air remains in the lungs, defined as the residual volume. This rapid and forceful exhalation of air generates forced vital capacity (FVC), or the largest volume of air that can be exhaled from the lungs, not including the residual volume left behind. Tracings obtained from this inhalation and exhalation during spirometry form the flow-volume loop, a graphical representation of lung function that can be useful as a diagnostic metric (**Fig. 1**).

The volume of air that can be exhaled forcefully in the first second of exhalation is known as the forced expiratory volume-first second (FEV_1), and is the most widely used parameter in measuring the mechanical properties of the lungs. In normal individuals, the FEV_1 represents about 75% to 85% of the FVC and the ratio of these 2 volumes can assist in differentiating obstructive from restrictive diseases. Lower FEV_1 values indicate more significant obstructive lung disease. In asthma, the FVC is generally conserved and is near normal whereas the FEV_1 is reduced. This reduced FEV_1/FVC ratio is characteristic of the patient with asthma.

Spirometry is often performed both before and after bronchodilator use to assess reversibility of airway obstruction. In this procedure, after the standard spirometry is completed, in the case of an abnormally reduced FEV_1, a short-acting β-2 agonist such as albuterol is administered via inhaler and the test repeated after several minutes. In patients with asthma, which is characterized by a reversible airway obstruction, the FEV_1 generally improves. Improvement of the FEV_1 by 12% or greater is generally diagnostic of asthma.

Spirometry values are based on referenced norms according to patient age, gender, race, height, and weight. This information is entered into the spirometer before conducting the test. As with peak flow meters, the accuracy of the test results is highly dependent on patient effort during the test. Therefore proper coaching throughout the test is essential to obtain maximal effort and results (**Table 1**). The patient is instructed to take a deep breath and blow out as hard and fast as possible and to take in a deep breath so to complete the flow-volume loop. The patient performs 3 tests or blows to get the best results (**Fig. 2**).

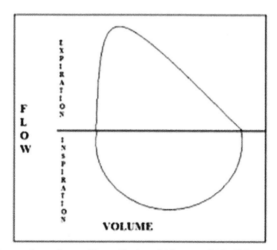

Fig. 1. Normal flow-volume loop. (*From* National Library of Medicine. Available at: http://openi.nlm.nih.gov/detailedresult.php?img=1297597_cc3516-6&req=4. Accessed September 6, 2013.)

Table 1
Questions to ask before baseline spirometry testing

How are you feeling today?	If the person has acute respiratory symptoms or illness, postpone testing for 3–5 d
Have you smoked any cigarettes, cigars, or pipes (including hookah/argileh) within the past hour?	If yes, postpone testing for 1 h
Have you used any inhaled medications within the past hour?	If yes, postpone testing for 1 h
Have you had any surgery in the past 4 wk (specifically abdominal; eye surgery; oral surgery)?	Cancel test and do not reschedule at this time

Bronchoprovocation

In patients with suspected asthma who have normal spirometry, testing is often done by stimulation of the airways with a bronchoconstrictive agent to assess the degree of bronchial hyperreactivity. Patients with mild asthma often have underlying subacute bronchial irritability and respond with a decline in FEV_1 during inhalational challenge with a bronchoconstrictor. Methacholine and histamine are the most commonly used agents for inhalational challenge, although methacholine is more widely used. It is considered safe and free from systemic side effects.

In performing inhalational challenges, increasing concentrations of methacholine are administered via a dosimeter through aerosolized inhalation. Five increasing

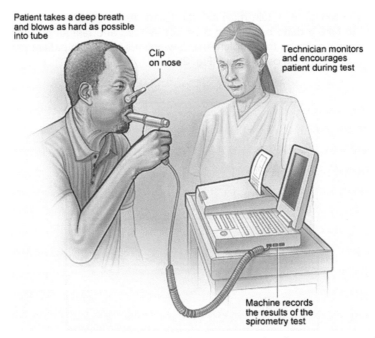

Fig. 2. Typical performance of spirometry. (*From* NIH, National Heart, Lung and Blood Institute. Available at: http://www.nhlbi.nih.gov/health/health-topics/topics/lft/types.html. Accessed July 3, 2013.)

concentrations are generally used. When there is a 20% drop in FEV_1 to inhalation, the test is terminated and is considered to be a positive indication of clinically significant airway hyperreactivity. The dosage required to trigger this reduction is known as the PC_{20FEV1}. If the FEV_1 does not drop by 20% at the highest concentration, then the test is considered negative. A PC_{20FEV1} of less than 8 mg/mL is interpreted as demonstrating clinically important airway hyperreactivity and would suggest a diagnosis of asthma.

Diffusing Capacity

Various pulmonary diseases can affect the ability of oxygen to diffuse from the alveolus into the capillary system in the lungs. Diseases that affect the lung parenchyma such as emphysema and cystic fibrosis can result in thickened alveolar-capillary membranes and impair air exchange. These findings are not generally seen in asthma, and diffusing capacity is not a commonly required test in patients suspected of having asthma.

Lung Volume

Lung volume measurements can be obtained to assess the total capacity of the lungs, which represents the full volume of the lungs, including the residual air remaining after forced expiration. Calculation of total capacity may be important in assessing restrictive lung diseases but is not generally necessary in the diagnosis and management of asthma.

SUMMARY

PFT is an important diagnostic modality in the workup of patients suspected of having asthma. It is also valuable to follow response to treatment among patients initiated and sustained on asthma therapy, and to assess patients complaining of symptoms suggestive of an asthma exacerbation. Spirometry is the most useful test in patients suspected of having asthma, and can easily be performed and interpreted in the otolaryngology office with readily available, inexpensive equipment. PFT should be considered for use in all otolaryngology patients with significant rhinitis and in those suspected of having lower respiratory disease.

REFERENCE

1. National Heart, Lung and Blood Institute. Expert Panel Report 3 (EPR3): guidelines for the diagnosis and management of asthma. Bethesda (MD): NHLBI; 2007.

Interpreting Spirometry: The Basics

Michael J. Parker, MD

KEYWORDS

- Spirometry • Airway • Asthma • Asthma diagnosis
- Objective monitoring of asthma therapy

KEY POINTS

- Spirometry is useful in detecting and monitoring airway disease in patients with symptoms, risk factors or suspicion of airway disease.
- Spirometry should accurately measure forced expiratory volume in 1 second, forced vital capacity, or forced expiratory volume in 6 seconds, and it should be reported both as the absolute measurement and as a percentage of normative data.
- Spirometry should be used to diagnose disease as well as monitor response to therapy and progression of disease over time.
- The contour of the flow-volume loop provides additional information with regard to the location of obstruction.
- Most patients with the suspicion of, or being treated for, asthma should have a baseline spirometry test.

INTRODUCTION

The classic signs and symptoms of asthma, which include intermittent dyspnea, cough, and wheezing, are often nonspecific, making it difficult to distinguish asthma from other respiratory diseases. The intermittent nature of the disease also makes it difficult for both patient and clinician to monitor the efficacy of therapy. Tests of airflow limitation are critical tools in the diagnosis and monitoring of asthma. Office spirometry is the most frequently used basic tool used to detect, confirm, and monitor obstructive airway disease (eg, asthma, chronic obstructive pulmonary disease [COPD]).[1,2] Spirometry plays an essential role in the management of patients with, or at risk for, respiratory dysfunction. Spirometry, in which a maximal inhalation is followed by a rapid and forceful complete exhalation into a spirometer, includes measurement of forced expiratory volume in the first second of expiration (FEV_1), forced vital capacity (FVC), and the relation of these two numbers (FEV_1/FVC) and the representation of the effort graphically as a flow-volume loop and volume-time graph. These measurements provide information that is essential to the diagnosis and management of asthma.[3]

Center For Sinus and Allergy Care, SUNY Upstate Medical University, 5639 West Genesee Street, Camillus, NY 13031, USA
E-mail address: mjparker.md@gmail.com

Otolaryngol Clin N Am 47 (2014) 39–53
http://dx.doi.org/10.1016/j.otc.2013.10.002
0030-6665/14/$ – see front matter © 2014 Elsevier Inc. All rights reserved.

This article discusses the use of spirometry in the office setting and discusses the primary measurements obtained and techniques used to obtain an accurate test. Issues related to equipment, performance of the forced expiratory maneuver, and interpretation of the data to obtain reliable and clinically useful information are discussed.[4–6] Examples of normal spirometric data as well as spirometric data from disease states are briefly reviewed.

INDICATIONS: WHO SHOULD BE TESTED?

Spirometry is an invaluable tool as a screening test of general respiratory health in the same way that blood pressure monitoring provides important information about the general health of the cardiovascular system.[7] Data from spirometry are also important to help convince patients with asthma to be more attentive to their disease, particularly those patients with mild intermittent asthma, who often have accommodated to their disease by modifying their lifestyles and avoiding situations that might provoke symptoms. Spirometry lends objectivity to subjective symptoms, is used to determine control in treated patients, and can be a tool to convince patients to be more compliant. It is a simple validated tool, with the ability to be used in nearly any setting.

SPIROMETRY MEASUREMENTS

Spirometry records the forced airflow from fully inflated lungs. Spirometry includes measurement of the FVC, the amount of air exhaled from the lungs from a maximal inhalation to a maximal exhalation, and the FEV_1. Both FEV_1 (airflow) and FVC (air volume) can be compromised by airway narrowing, inflammatory and bronchospastic factors, and mucus plugging, which can obstruct or occlude some of the small (or even larger) airways. These values are typically reported in 2 ways: as a volume measurement (milliliters or liters of air), or as a percentage of the predicted normative or expected value for that patient's age, height, gender, and race from data obtained in the National Health and Nutrition Examination Survey III (NHANES III).[8]

The FEV_1 is the most important spirometric measurement for assessment of the severity of airflow obstruction. The highest FEV_1 from the 3 acceptable forced expiratory maneuvers is used for interpretation, even if it does not come from the maneuver with the highest FVC.[7]

In patients with asthma, the FEV_1 declines are in direct and linear proportion with clinical worsening of airway obstruction. FEV_1 has been shown to increase with successful treatment of airway obstruction. The FEV_1 should be used to determine the degree of obstruction (mild, moderate, or severe) and for serial comparisons when following patients with asthma.[3] The measured FEV_1 is usually expressed as a percentage of the predicted value for determination of normality. The reference values from the NHANES III study (recently expanded to preschool children) are recommended for use throughout North America.[9,10] The lower limit of normal FEV_1 is more accurately defined by the fifth percentile of healthy never-smokers, instead of the traditional 80% of predicted.[11]

The FVC (also known as the forced expiratory volume) is the maximal volume of air exhaled with a maximally forced effort from a position of full inspiration and is expressed in liters. The highest FVC from the 3 acceptable forced expiratory maneuvers is used for interpretation.[8]

The FVC may be reduced by suboptimal patient effort, airflow limitation, restriction (eg, from lung parenchymal, pleural, or thoracic cage disease), or a combination of these. In general, a moderately or severely low FVC needs further evaluation with a more complete battery of pulmonary function tests.[12]

The forced expiratory volume in 6 seconds (FEV_6) is a term that is sometimes used to describe the forced expiratory volume in 6 seconds of maximal exhalation, obtained by stopping the expiratory effort after 6 seconds rather than at cessation of airflow. This surrogate for the FVC is acceptable.[12–15] The advantages of the FEV_6 compared with FVC include less frustration by the patient after repeated attempts at a prolonged and forceful blow and by the technician trying to achieve an end-of-test plateau. Additional advantages of an FEV_6 compared with the FVC include a smaller chance of syncope, shorter testing time, and better repeatability, without loss of sensitivity or specificity.

Together, the FEV_1 and FVC (or FEV_6) are considered the most readily available and most useful components of spirometry and the most reflective of an obstructive disease state such as asthma.

Another important relationship shown by spirometry is the ratio between the FEV_1 and FVC: the FEV_1/FVC ratio is the fraction of FVC that can be exhaled in the first second. It is the most important parameter for detecting airflow limitation in diseases like asthma. However, once established, the ratio has little value in predicting progression of disease because typically both the FVC and FEV_1 decline with progression of disease. The threshold for an abnormal FEV_1/FVC ratio is the fifth percentile lower limit of normal.[16]

Additional lung functions that can be measured during spirometry include the forced expiratory flow of the midexpiratory phase of forced expiration. This middle 50% of the total FVC is called the forced expiratory flow 25% to 75% ($FEF_{25\%–75\%}$), and has been thought to reflect the reactivity in the mid to small airway. Although asthma is a disease of the small to midsized airway, the clinical value of this value as a single meaningful number has recently been questioned. Although of use in the overall picture of airway reactivity, therapeutic decisions should not be based exclusively on this number.[8]

GRAPHIC REPRESENTATION OF DATA
Flow-Volume Loops

This approach to the data yields useful additional information beyond that obtained by analysis of FEV_1 and FVC measurements.[16,17] Information generated during the office spirometry can be analyzed by plotting the data, creating a graph of the test known as the flow-volume loop (also called a spirogram). The flow-volume relationship or loop is created by plotting flow against volume during the FVC (forced expiratory) maneuver. The flow-volume loop is a plot of inspiratory and expiratory flow in liters per second (on the y-axis) against volume (on the x-axis) during the performance of maximally forced inspiratory and expiratory maneuvers (**Fig. 1**). Analysis of this loop provides rapidly recognizable patterns that permit the clinician to differentiate bronchial asthma from airflow limitations with other causes, such as vocal cord dysfunction or a fixed obstruction. The flow-volume loop can also show reversibility of the disease process, differentiate an obstructive pattern of airflow from a restrictive pattern, and easily separates a quality maximal effort from a suboptimal test.

The normal expiratory portion of a well-performed flow-volume loop is characterized by a rapid increase to the peak flow rate, followed by a nearly linear decrease in flow as the patient exhales toward residual volume. Less-than-optimal effort, early glottic closure, and coughing are some of the variables that can influence the expiratory curve (**Figs. 2–4**). The expiratory curve should be examined on every test as a key component of the test interpretation.

In contrast, the inspiratory curve is a symmetric, saddle-shaped curve. The flow rate at the midpoint of exhalation (between total lung capacity and residual volume) is normally approximately equivalent to the flow rate at the midpoint of inspiration.

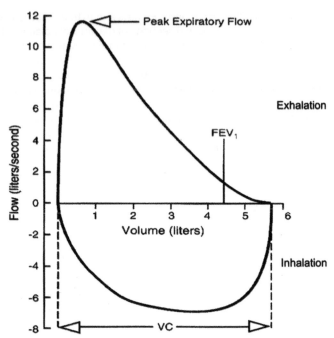

Fig. 1. Normal flow-volume loop. Expiratory flow above the x-axis, inspiratory flow below the x-axis. Note the closed nature of the loop, indicating no air leak with all air flow measured by the spirometer. Near-vertical increase in the forced expiratory flow, followed by a near-linear decline. The shapes of both the inspiratory and expiratory curves are useful in understanding the test parameters. VC, vital capacity. (*From* Crapo RO. Pulmonary-function testing. N Engl J Med 1994;331:28; with permission.)

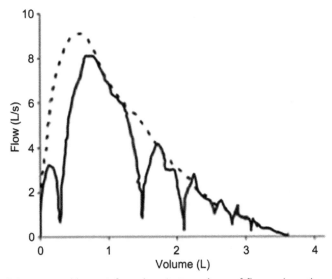

Fig. 2. Cough interrupted loop. A forced expiratory phase of flow-volume loop resulting in less than optimal test results secondary to a coughing during the test. When possible, this effort should be repeated. (*From* Townsend MC. Spirometry in the occupational health setting—2011 update. J Occup Env 2011;53(5):569–84; with permission.)

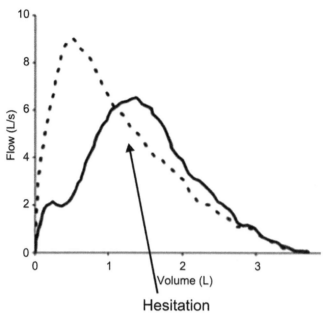

Hesitation

Fig. 3. Poor-quality flow-volume loop related to some hesitation (or stuttering) to the start of the effort is unacceptable. (*From* Townsend MC. Spirometry in the occupational health setting—2011 update. J Occup Env 2011;53(5):569–84; with permission.)

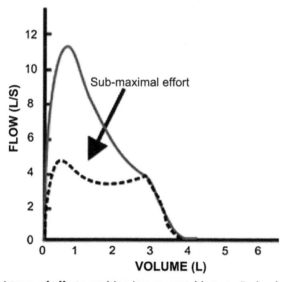

Fig. 4. Poor consistency of efforts resulting in unacceptable tests. Each subsequent maximal effort should be inspected and overlaid on previous efforts. Quality data (repeated maximal efforts) should result in nearly superimposed images. (*From* Centers for Disease Control and Prevention. Spirometry quality assurance: common errors and their impact on test results. Available at: http://www.cdc.gov/niosh/docs/2012-116/pdfs/2012-116.pdf. Accessed October 8, 2013.)

Changes in the contour of the loop can aid in the diagnosis, type, and localization of airway disease and are critical components of spirometry interpretation.[11] Characteristic flow-volume loop patterns are also often found in certain forms of restrictive disease, although flow-volume studies are not considered primary diagnostic aids in the evaluation of these disorders.

A flow-volume loop representative of an obstructive disorder (asthma, COPD) typically shows a departure from the linear slope of the flow curve and instead is a scalloped or scooped-out concavity (**Fig. 5**). Lung volumes are typically normal in isolated obstructive disease.

A restrictive pattern as shown by a flow-volume loop reflects diminished lung volume and maintains a linear slope to the flow curve (**Fig. 6**). Patients occasionally show a mixed pattern producing a flow-volume loop that has characteristics of both an obstructive (concavity) and restrictive pattern (diminished volume) (**Fig. 7**).

The flow-volume loop can also show areas of obstruction of airflow not related to the small and midsized airway. Examples include fixed upper airway obstruction (**Fig. 8**),

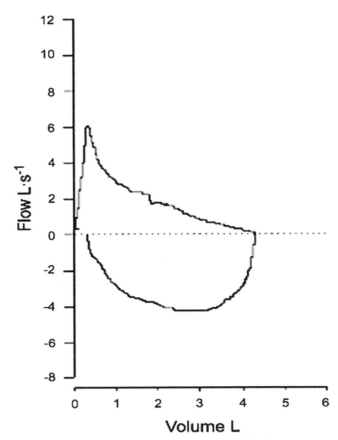

Fig. 5. Moderate obstructive pattern of flow-volume loop. The forced expiratory curve of the flow-volume loop (above the x-axis) shows a concavity or scalloping of the normally linear sloped portion of the curve. The inspiratory tracing (below the x-axis) is normal. There is no significant decrease in lung volume. (*From* Miller MR, Hankinson J, Brusasco V, et al. Standardisation of spirometry. Eur Respir J 2005;26:319–38; with permission.)

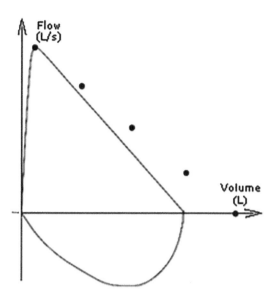

Fig. 6. Restrictive pattern of flow-volume loop. A diminished volume (x-axis) typifies a flow-volume loop showing a restrictive pattern. The descending arm of the expiratory loop typically remains linear, without the concavity seen in an obstructive pattern. (*From* Spirométrie Info. Interpretation of the flow-volume loop. Available at: http://www.spirometrie.info/fvc. html. Accessed October 8, 2013; with permission.)

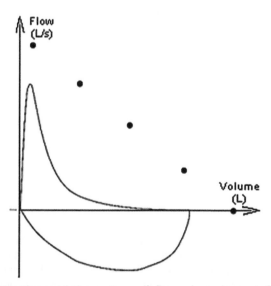

Fig. 7. Mixed obstructive-restrictive pattern of flow-volume loop. A flow-volume loop showing both the concave characteristics of an obstructive pattern on the descending limb of the expiratory loop, combined with reduced volume along the horizontal axis. (*From* Spirométrie Info. Interpretation of the flow-volume loop. Available at: http://www. spirometrie.info/fvc.html. Accessed October 8, 2013; with permission.)

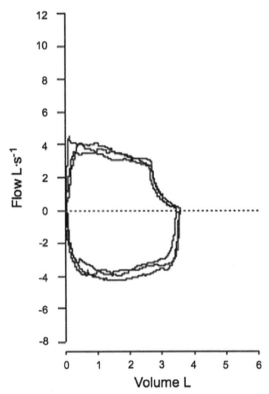

Fig. 8. Fixed upper airway obstruction. (*From* Miller MR, Hankinson J, Brusasco V, et al. Standardisation of spirometry. Eur Respir J 2005;26:319–38; with permission.)

variable intrathoracic obstruction (**Fig. 9**), variable extrathoracic obstruction (**Fig. 10**), and vocal cord dysfunction.

Volume-Time Graph

Although generally thought to be less important than the flow-volume loop, the volume-time graph plots the volume (in liters) of a maximal forced expiration on the y-axis and time (in seconds) along the x-axis. The volume-time tracing shows the FEV_1 well and can be used to quickly evaluate the effort of the test and the FEV_1 (**Fig. 11**) and to show declines in FEV_1.

Equipment

There has been a significant improvement in the availability and quality of office spirometers over the last 2 decades, with the introduction of flow-sensing turbine spirometers and pneumotachographs replacing the volume-displacement spirometer. Most spirometers manufactured since 1990 are accurate, although some of the flow-sensing office spirometers can produce falsely increased FVC and FEV_1, suggesting greater attention to routine calibration.[18] In general, the spirometric equipment can be purchased for roughly US$2000, takes up little space, and should be able to be integrated with the patients Electronic Health Record. Guidelines published by the National Lung Health Education Program have suggested a list of required features (eg, graphic output).[19]

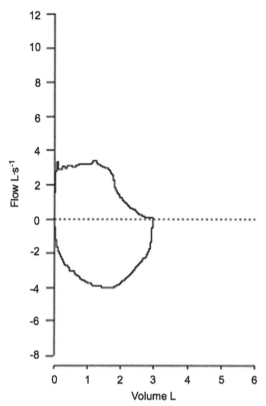

Fig. 9. Variable intrathoracic airway obstruction. (*From* Miller MR, Hankinson J, Brusasco V, et al. Standardisation of spirometry. Eur Respir J 2005;26:319–38; with permission.)

As with any reusable medical device, the risk of cross-contamination between patients needs to be considered and single-use disposable flow sensors are preferable, because they greatly reduce the risk of inhalation cross-contamination.

Quality Control/Calibration

Office spirometers are designed with internal calibration algorithms that are routinely performed internally by the device. Spirometers should accurately measure the FEV_1, FEV_6, and FVC, and also provide quality checks and error messages. In addition to the internal calibration algorithms in the spirometer, office practices using spirometers should involve daily calibration checks. These checks are typically performed using a 3-L syringe that is filled with air and is then discharged into the spirometer via the mouthpiece 3 times, allowing the unit to measure the average of a standard volume. The volumes read by the machine should be within 3.5% of 3 L. If the spirometer reading remains outside these limits after replacing the flow sensor, the device should be removed from use until checked by the manufacturer.[10]

Patient Participation/Contraindications

A potential challenge of spirometry is that it requires active patient participation to produce accurate and reproducible data. Spirometry is also generally considered safe but at times requires vigorous efforts, so appropriate but specific contraindications exist

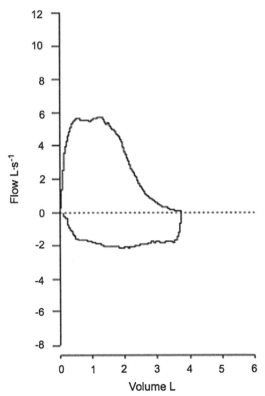

Fig. 10. Variable extrathoracic airway obstruction. (*From* Miller MR, Hankinson J, Brusasco V, et al. Standardisation of spirometry. Eur Respir J 2005;26:319–38; with permission.)

and include a history of a myocardial infarction within the last month, unstable angina, recent thoracoabdominal surgery, recent ophthalmic surgery, thoracic or abdominal aneurysm, or current pneumothorax.[20] Spirometry is effort dependent and therefore patient cooperation and understanding while performing the test is essential in obtaining optimal results.

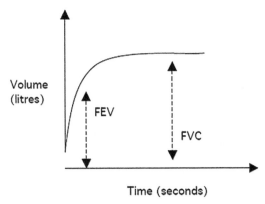

Fig. 11. Normal volume-time graph. FEV, forced expiratory volume. (*From* Ranu H, Wilde M, Madden B. Pulmonary function tests. Ulster Med J 2011;80(2):84–90; with permission.)

Procedure

Patients are typically tested in a private (confidential) area that is at a comfortable temperature, with adequate lighting, without distractions, and with a sink nearby for hand washing. Patients are usually seated in a chair without wheels during spirometry to prevent the risk of injury from falling during a syncopal event. To prevent air leakage through the nasal passages during the procedure, a nose clip or manual occlusion of the nares can be helpful, although adequate test results can be obtained without nasal occlusion.[8] Patients are instructed to take a deep/maximal inhalation before placing the mouthpiece in their mouths. Immediately after the deep inhalation, the mouthpiece is placed just inside the mouth, between the teeth, sealing the lips tightly around the mouthpiece to prevent air leakage during the test. Patients are instructed to exhale or blast the air out of their lungs into the mouthpiece. Exhalation should last for at least 6 seconds.

Three separate maneuvers are usually performed to ensure that each effort is reproducible (less than 200 mL variation) and accurate. Patients are allowed to rest and catch their breath between each procedure. The quality of the tests should be reviewed and additional tests may be needed if one or more of the flow-volume curves are unacceptable.

A key feature of spirometry is the concept of a maximal effort, requiring patient participation in the process. Suboptimal efforts provide unreliable results and may lead to inaccurate diagnosis or poor disease management. Poor initiation or hesitation of blast, exhalation cough, suboptimal effort, early cessation of effort, and variability of effort can all be identified on the flow-volume loop and should prompt a repeat attempt with patient coaching.

Patient Data Entry/"Normative" Data

Because data are recorded and compared with normative data, it is essential that the nurse or technician enter correct values for age, height, gender, and ethnicity. These values are used to generate the appropriate predicted values for each individual patient.[10,21] Percent predicted values that are higher or lower than expected are a clue that an incorrect age or height value may have been entered. Weight and waist circumference should also be measured because abdominal obesity is a common cause of a mildly low FVC and a restrictive pattern of lung disease on spirograms.[22]

Office Personnel/Patient Instruction/Encouragement

An important task of the nurse or technician supervising the procedure is to obtain a maximal effort and reproducible data from the patient. Even with the use of accurate instruments, office spirometry results may be misleading if the patient's efforts are submaximal. Unlike most other medical tests in which the patient remains passive, accurate spirometry results require significant exertion on the part of the patient. The technician must instruct and encourage the patient to perform the breathing maneuvers. The effort is typically broken down into 3 phases of instruction and coaching during the maneuver. The patient is first coached to take as deep a breath as possible, followed by loud vocal encouragement from the nurse or technician to blast out the air into the spirometer. The encouragement continues with the prompting and support to continue the exhaling for at least 6 seconds. Acceptable tests usually include a satisfactory start of exhalation, no cough or glottal closure, no evidence of a leak, no early termination, and a satisfactory exhalation (6 seconds).

Test Adequacy

Spirometry requires active and vigorous patient participation to produce a maximal forceful exhalation of full vital capacity of the lungs. Factors that affect test accuracy include the ability of the patient to follow instructions and/or be capable of performing the forceful exhalation, coaching from the technologists, the accuracy and calibration of the spirometer, and the interpretation of the results. An adequate test usually requires 3 acceptable and reproducible FVC maneuvers. The clinician and technician must learn to recognize the patterns of acceptable and unacceptable efforts, because poorly performed maneuvers often mimic disease patterns. Detection of poorly performed maneuvers requires direct inspection of both flow-volume curves and volume-time spirograms.[8,10] An acceptable maneuver requires a sharp peak in the flow curve and an expiratory duration greater than 6 seconds. Two, and preferably 3, acceptable maneuvers should be available for analysis.

Reproducibility is determined by comparing the flow-volume loops and by comparing the FVC values of the maneuvers. Adequate spirometry should generate flow-volume loops that, when superimposed on one another, are nearly indistinguishable from each other. With regard to the FVC, the 2 highest values for FVC should be within 0.15 L of each other.[8,9] The 2 highest values for FEV_1 should similarly be within 0.15 L of each other.

Interpretation

General principles used to interpret the test include examination of the curve, examination of the FEV_1/FVC, and then examination of the FEV_1 and the $FEF_{25\%-75\%}$. All tracings from the forced expiratory maneuvers (flow-volume loop and volume-time graph) should be examined for acceptability and reproducibility, according to criteria mentioned earlier. The study should then be classified as normal, borderline, or abnormal, an abnormal study showing either an obstructive, restrictive, or mixed pattern (see **Figs. 5–7**). The severity of any obstructive impairment is then assessed using the FEV_1/FVC and FEV_1 data (**Box 1**).

Healthy patients expire approximately 80% of the air from their lungs in the first second during the FVC maneuver. A patient with an obstruction of the upper airways has a diminished FEV_1/FVC. An FEV_1/FVC that is too high suggests a restriction of the pulmonary volume (diminished FVC).

An approach to the interpretation of abnormal values is provided (see **Box 1**).[19] The specific values assigned to mild, moderate, and severe disease vary among the different guidelines.[9]

Postbronchodilator Spirometry

Airflow limitation from asthma typically shows some degree of reversibility following acute treatment with a beta-agonist. The currently recommended criteria for a significant response to a bronchodilator in adults are an increase in FVC or FEV_1 by 12% (and by at least 200 mL).[23]

In preparation for assessing bronchodilator reversibility, short-acting inhaled bronchodilators (eg, albuterol, salbutamol, ipratropium) should not be used for up to 4 hours before testing.[8] Long-acting beta-agonist bronchodilators (eg, salmeterol, formoterol) should be omitted for 12 hours before testing, and the long-acting anticholinergic agent tiotropium is omitted for 24 hours. Most laboratories use 2 metered-dose inhaler inhalations of a rapidly acting beta-agonist, such as albuterol, 108 mcg albuterol sulfate (90 mcg albuterol base) from mouthpiece per actuation, via a chamber with an appropriate delay (10–20 minutes) to allow the beta-agonist to work. A case can also be made for the administration of a beta-agonist by nebulizer until side effects, such as heart rate more than 150 beats per minute, are observed. This maximal approach eliminates issues of aerosol distribution, inadequate dose response, and

---

Box 1

Numeric Interpretation: Disease States and measured FEV₁ and FEV₁/FVC ratios

If the FEV_1/FVC ratio is normal and the FEV_1 is greater than 80% of predicted, then the spirometry is normal.

If the FEV_1/FVC ratio is reduced and the FEV_1 is less than 80% of predicted, then the spirometry is consistent with an obstructive pattern.

  FEV_1 80%–70% predicted = mild obstruction

  FEV_1 50%–69% predicted = moderate obstruction

  FEV_1<50% predicted = severe obstruction

If the FEV_1/FVC is reduced and the FEV_1 is greater than 80% predicted, spirometry may be normal; this finding may be caused by a prolonged exhalation phase leading to overestimation of the FVC.

If the FEV_1/FVC ratio is normal, but the FVC is mildly reduced (70%–80% predicted), the cause may be abdominal obesity or poor technique.

If the FEV_1/FVC ratio is normal, but the FVC is less than 80% of predicted, consider referring the patient to a pulmonary function laboratory for measurement of lung volumes and diffusing capacity (carbon monoxide diffusion in the lung) to assess for a possible restrictive lung disease (eg, interstitial lung disease or respiratory muscle weakness).

Adapted from Pellegrino R, Viegi G, Brusasco V, et al. Interpretative strategies for lung function tests. Eur Respir J 2005;26:948–68.

---

patient technique, which can be minimized with the use of a spacer/chamber.[24] The prebronchodilator and postbronchodilator data are compared to assess for the presence of reversible air flow obstruction (**Fig. 12**). In patients with baseline airflow limitation, failure to improve following bronchodilator administration suggests an alternate

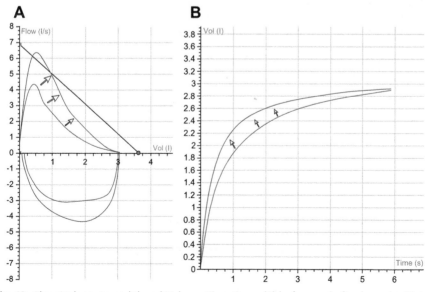

Fig. 12. Flow-Volume Loop (*A*) and Volume-Time Curve (*B*) before and after bronchodilator. *Pink line* indicates pre-bronchodilator. *Red line* indicates post-bronchodilator. The *arrows* indicate the change in flow from bronchodilator.

diagnosis (eg, COPD) or airway inflammation that requires additional therapy (eg, glucocorticoids). In patients with normal spirometry at baseline, a bronchodilator response with an increase in FEV_1 of more than 8% may suggest underlying airflow limitation, because the patient may have once had higher than predicted lung function.[23–25]

Bronchoprovocation Challenge

In patients with a history consistent with intermittent asthma and normal spirometric data, strategies should be considered to confirm or refute the diagnosis of asthma. These patients sometimes present with no airflow limitation on spirometry and may not show reversal/improvement after bronchodilator administration. In such patients, a bronchial challenge (eg, methacholine challenge, exercise challenge test) is indicated to show reversible airflow obstruction that can be provoked. A discussion of methacholine inhalation challenge and other types of bronchoprovocation tests is beyond the scope of this article.

SUMMARY

Spirometry is useful to detect and monitor airway disease in patients with symptoms, risk factors, or suspicion of airway disease. Spirometric equipment is readily available and requires little maintenance and some calibration.

Acceptable tests require active patient participation and coaching. At least 3 quality maneuvers should be preformed. Clinician and technician must learn to recognize the patterns of an unacceptable test effort.

Spirometry should accurately measure FEV_1, FVC (or FEV_6), and it should be reported as both an absolute measurement and as a percentage of normative data. The FEV_1/FVC ratio is important for distinguishing obstructive from restrictive airway disease. Spirometry should be used to diagnose disease as well as monitor response to therapy and progression of disease over time.

The flow-volume loop is a plot of inspiratory and expiratory flow against volume. The shape of the flow-volume loop in asthma and obstructive lung disease typically shows a scooped-out or concave upward pattern. The contour of the flow-volume loop provides additional information with regard to the location of obstruction.

Almost all patients with the suspicion of, or being treated for, asthma should have a baseline spirometry test. The test should be repeated at least annually in asthmatic patients as needed to manage and monitor the disease.

REFERENCES

1. Enright P, Quanjer P. Don't diagnose mild COPD without confirming airway obstruction after an inhaled bronchodilator. COPD 2007;4:89.
2. Lin K, Watkins B, Johnson T, et al. Screening for chronic obstructive pulmonary disease using spirometry: summary of the evidence for the U.S. Preventive Services Task Force. Ann Intern Med 2008;148:535.
3. National Asthma Education and Prevention Program: expert panel report III: guidelines for the diagnosis and management of asthma. Bethesda (MD): National Heart, Lung, and Blood Institute; 2007. NIH publication no. 08-4051. Available at: http://www.nhlbi.nih.gov/guidelines/asthma/asthgdln.htm. Accessed January 5, 2013.
4. Enright PL, Studnicka M, Zielinski J. Spirometry to detect and manage COPD and asthma in the primary care setting. Eur Respir Mon 2005;31:1.

5. Walters JA, Hansen EC, Johns DP, et al. A mixed methods study to compare models of spirometry delivery in primary care for patients at risk of COPD. Thorax 2008;63:408.

6. Lusuardi M, De Benedetto F, Paggiaro P, et al. A randomized controlled trial on office spirometry in asthma and COPD in standard general practice: data from spirometry in asthma and COPD: a comparative evaluation Italian study. Chest 2006;129:844.

7. Miller MR, Hankinson J, Brusasco V, et al. Standardisation of spirometry. Eur Respir J 2005;26:319.

8. Hankinson JL, Odencrantz JR, Fedan KB. Spirometric reference values from a sample of the general U.S. population. Am J Respir Crit Care Med 1999;159:179.

9. Pellegrino R, Viegi G, Brusasco V, et al. Interpretative strategies for lung function tests. Eur Respir J 2005;26:948.

10. Stanojevic S, Wade A, Stocks J, et al. Reference ranges for spirometry across all ages: a new approach. Am J Respir Crit Care Med 2008;177:253.

11. Miller MR, Quanjer PH, Swanney MP, et al. Interpreting lung function data using 80% predicted and fixed thresholds misclassifies more than 20% of patients. Chest 2011;139:52.

12. Vandervoorde J, Verbanck S, Shuermans D, et al. Forced vital capacity and forced expiratory volume in six seconds as predictors of reduced total lung capacity. Eur Respir J 2008;31:391.

13. Swanney MP, Jensen RL, Crichton DA, et al. FEV(6) is an acceptable surrogate for FVC in the spirometric diagnosis of airway obstruction and restriction. Am J Respir Crit Care Med 2000;162:917.

14. Demir T, Ikitimur HD, Koc N, et al. The role of FEV6 in the detection of airway obstruction. Respir Med 2005;99:103.

15. Vandevoorde J, Verbanck S, Schuermans D, et al. FEV1/FEV6 and FEV6 as an alternative for FEV1/FVC and FVC in the spirometric detection of airway obstruction and restriction. Chest 2005;127:1560.

16. Irvin CG. Development, structure, and physiology in normal and asthmatic lung. In: Adkinson NF Jr, editor. Middleton's allergy principles and practice. 8th edition. St Louis (MO): Elsevier; 2013. p. 709–10.

17. Crapo RO. Pulmonary-function testing. N Engl J Med 1994;331:25.

18. Schermer TR, Verweij EH, Cretier R, et al. Accuracy and precision of desktop spirometers in general practice. Respiration 2012;83:344.

19. Ferguson GT, Enright PL, Buist AS, et al. Office spirometry for lung health assessment in adults: a consensus statement from the National Lung Health Education Program. Chest 2000;117:1146.

20. Ranu H, Wilde M, Madden B. Pulmonary function tests. Ulster Med J 2011;80(2):84–90.

21. Available at: http://www.cdc.gov/nchs/nhanes/about_nhanes.htm. Accessed May 10, 2013.

22. Leone N, Courbon D, Thomas F, et al. Lung function impairment and metabolic syndrome: the critical role of abdominal obesity. Am J Respir Crit Care Med 2009;179:509.

23. Quadrelli SA, Roncoroni AJ, Montiel GC. Evaluation of bronchodilator response in patients with airway obstruction. Respir Med 1999;93:630.

24. Smith HR, Irvin CG, Cherniack RM. The utility of spirometry in the diagnosis of reversible airways obstruction. Chest 1992;101:1577.

25. Lung function testing: selection of reference values and interpretative strategies. American Thoracic Society. Am Rev Respir Dis 1991;144:1202.

Asthma Pharmacotherapy

Minka L. Schofield, MD

KEYWORDS

- Asthma • Therapy • Medications • Short acting beta agonists
- Inhaled corticosteroids • Long acting beta agonists • Anti-IgE therapy

KEY POINTS

- Inhaled SABAs are the preferred medication for intermittent asthma symptoms and acute reversal of bronchoconstriction.
- Persistent asthma symptoms are preferably managed with inhaled corticosteroids (ICSs) with or without adjunctive therapy consisting of LTRAs, zileuton, or theophylline.
- Particle size of inhalers plays a key role in lung deposition and hence effectiveness.
- Omalizumab, anti-IgE therapy injection, has been indicated as an adjunct for persistent allergic patients with asthma uncontrolled with ICS+LABA combination therapy with a low risk of anaphylaxis after injection.
- Many novel asthma therapies are being investigated that target gene expression, anti-inflammatory mechanisms, and steroid resistance.

INTRODUCTION

Asthma represents a chronic inflammatory process marked by bronchial hyperactivity, mucus hypersecretion, and airway edema that leads to airway obstruction. These changes in the airway initially are reversible, but with continued airway remodeling the extent of reversibility may vary, leading to more difficult management. The goals of asthma pharmacotherapy are to reverse the inflammatory state and airway obstruction. The National Asthma Education and Prevention Program (NAEPP) Expert Panel has devised evidence-based guidelines for asthma care, including recommendations for therapy based on asthma severity (**Fig. 1**).[1]

BETA-2 AGONISTS
Short-Acting Beta-2 Agonists

Short-acting beta-2 agonists (SABAs), such as albuterol and levalbuterol, are recommended for intermittent asthma symptoms and serve to immediately reverse

---

Disclosures: None.
Division of Sinus and Allergy, Department of Otolaryngology-Head and Neck Surgery, The Eye and Ear Institute, Wexner Medical Center, The Ohio State University, 915 Olentangy River Road, Suite 4000, Columbus, OH 43212, USA
E-mail address: minka.schofield@osumc.edu

Otolaryngol Clin N Am 47 (2014) 55–64
http://dx.doi.org/10.1016/j.otc.2013.09.011
0030-6665/14/$ – see front matter © 2014 Elsevier Inc. All rights reserved.

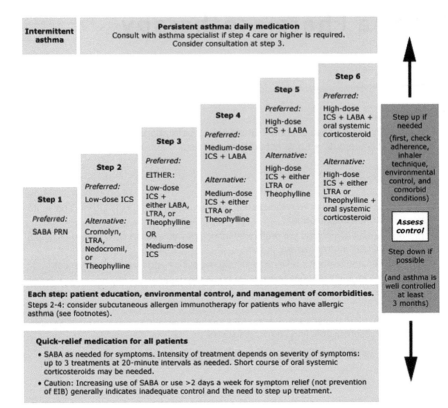

Fig. 1. NAEPP expert panel guidelines for asthma care. (*From* National Heart, Lung, and Blood Institute. Full Report 2007, guidelines for the diagnosis and management of asthma. Available at: www.nhlbi.nih.gov/guidelines/asthma. Accessed September 10, 2013.)

bronchoconstriction via potent bronchodilation. The mechanism of action is via a selective interaction on beta-2 receptors of bronchial smooth muscle to achieve bronchodilation. SABAs are the preferred medication for acute asthma exacerbations as a rescue inhaler due to the quick onset of bronchodilation. Regular use of SABAs is not recommended because of the development of tachyphylaxis and increased hyper responsiveness.

Long-Acting Beta-2 Agonists

Long-acting beta-2 agonists (LABAs), salmeterol and formoterol, provide approximately 12 hours of bronchodilation. The mechanism by which LABAs provide long-acting effects has not been clearly delineated. Multiple mechanisms have been described in the development of once-daily ultra- LABA preparations, including partitioning of the drug into lipophilic compartments after inhalation forming small depots of the drug, the presence of small lipid rafts in airway smooth muscle, and the tight binding to beta-2 adrenoreceptor and formation of ternary complexes.[2]

Since 2005, LABAs are no longer recommended as sole agents for the management of asthma. In 1993, Castle and colleagues,[3] in a study using salmeterol, showed convincing evidence that mortality increased threefold in patients with asthma, which led to a study influenced by the Food and Drug Administration (FDA), the Salmeterol

Multicentre Asthma Research Trial (SMART) study in 1996.[4] The study was aborted due to increased exacerbations and mortality. Subsequent studies using formoterol in higher doses demonstrated increased exacerbations as well.[5]

LABAs are currently recommended as a combination therapy with corticosteroids based on an FDA 2008 meta-analysis showing no significant safety risks.[6] Per NAEPP guidelines, the use of LABAs + inhaled corticosteroids (ICSs) is indicated in persistent asthma uncontrolled with ICSs alone. Three preparations are available: budesonide/formoterol, mometasone/formoterol, and fluticasone/salmeterol.

A 2011 meta-analysis comparing fluticasone/salmeterol with budesonide/formoterol showed no significant difference between the 2 preparations as it relates to oral steroid requirements, hospital admissions, rescue inhaler use, and lung function.[7] Another comparison study demonstrated that the odds of bronchodilation within 5 minutes was almost 4 times higher with fluticasone/formoterol over fluticasone/salmeterol, suggesting that this benefit may influence patient compliance with medication.[8] In an effort to manage patients with asthma using the lowest effective dose of ICS/LABA, Hojo and colleagues[9] proposed a step-down protocol to avoid asthma exacerbations. Patients were controlled on budesonide/formoterol at 640/18 µg (4 puffs/day) followed by step-down to 320/9 µg/day (2 puffs/day) when either the forced expired nitric oxide (FeNO) decreased to 28 or lower while the asthma control test (ACT) was 22 or higher or the ACT was 24 points or higher at 3 consecutive visits. After a 48-week study period, asthma control was stable based on SABA use and the number of acute exacerbations.

The selectivity of beta-2 agonists over alpha and beta-1 receptors results in fewer cardiac side effects, such as tachycardia and palpitations. Levalbuterol is an entamer of albuterol associated with even fewer cardiac side effects. Use of beta-2 agonists in diabetic patients is cautioned because of the risk of ketoacidosis related to induction of liver glycogenolysis via beta-adrenoreceptor. Other adverse reactions include hypokalemia, tremor, irritation, or anxiety after use.

ANTICHOLINERGICS

Anticholinergic agents, primarily ipratroprium, also function as bronchodilators by inhibiting the vagal muscarinic receptors on smooth muscle. These agents can be effective especially in patients who do not tolerate SABAs. Tiotropium, a long-acting antimuscarinic, has been shown to be an effective bronchodilator in chronic obstructive pulmonary disease (COPD) and investigators have also shown tiotropium to be effective in asthma. Kerstjens and colleagues[10] demonstrated in 2 randomized controlled trials that tiotropium improved asthma control in patients with poorly controlled asthma on ICSs and LABAs. Tiotropium was administered as 2 puffs of 2.5 µg via mist inhaler in addition to any previous asthma medications before the trial. After a 48-week trial period, the investigators observed an improvement in forced expiratory volume in 1 second (FEV1) in the first 24 weeks with an overall reduction in the risk of a severe exacerbation by 21% compared with placebo.

CORTICOSTEROIDS

The mechanism of action of corticosteroids is complex, involving cellular and molecular mechanisms having direct and indirect influences on the airway. In general, corticosteroids have been shown to enhance the beta-adrenergic response that relieves muscle spasm, reverse edema by decreasing vascular permeability and the inhibition of leukotriene C4 (LTC4) and LTD4, decrease mucus by inhibiting macrophage release of secretagogue, and inhibit chemotaxis to reverse inflammatory response.[11] The binding of glucocorticoid receptors triggers multiple genes involved in regulating airway inflammation (**Box 1**).[12]

ICS

ICSs have become the preferred long-term treatment recommendation for patients classified as having persistent asthma. Steroids are effective during the late phase

---

Box 1
Effect of corticosteroids on gene transcription

Increased transcription

Annexin-1 (lipocortin-1, phospholipase A_2 inhibitor)

Beta-2 adrenoceptors

Clara cell protein (CC10, phospholipase A_2 inhibitor)

Glucocorticoid-induced leucine zipper protein

IL-1 receptor antagonist

IL-1 receptor 2 (decoy receptor)

Inhibitor of NF-κB (IκB-α)

IL-10

Mitogen-activated protein kinase phosphatase-1

Secretory leukoprotease inhibitor

Decreased transcription

Cytokines

    IL-1, IL-2, IL-3, IL-4, IL-5, IL-6, IL-9, IL-11, IL-12, IL-13, IL-16, IL-17, IL-18, TNFα, GM-CSF, stem cell factor

Chemokines

    IL-8, RANTES, MIP-1α, MCP-1, MCP-3, MCP-4, eotaxins

Adhesion molecules

    E-selectin, ICAM-1, VCAM-1

Inflammatory enzymes

    Cytoplasmic phospholipase A_2

    Inducible cyclooxygenase (COX-2)

    Inducible nitric oxide synthase

Inflammatory receptors

    Bradykinin Beta-2 receptors

    Tachykinin NK_1-receptors, NK_2-receptors

Peptides

    Endothelin-1

Abbreviations: GM-CSF, granulocyte-macrophage colony stimulating factor; ICAM, intercellular adhesion molecule; IL, interleukin; MCP, monocyte chemoattractant protein; MIP, macrophage inflammatory protein; RANTES, released by normal activated T cells expressed and secreted; TNF, tumor necrosis factor; VCAM, vascular-endothelial cell adhesion molecule.
From Jang A. Steroid response in refractory asthmatics. Korean J Intern Med 2012;27:143–8; with permission.

of the hypersensitivity response; hence, are not indicated for acute reversal of bronchoconstriction during the immediate hypersensitivity reaction like SABAs. Instead, these agents function to decrease the inflammation and edema associated with asthma through continual use of the medication.

ICSs also have a direct anti-inflammatory effect on the airway, demonstrated in a study randomizing patients with asthma on placebo, oral steroid, and inhaled steroid.[13] The ICS group demonstrated better asthma control with no systemic steroid detected, suggesting that the anti-inflammatory effects of the ICS is direct or via topical effects on lung steroid receptors.

The effectiveness of these agents seems to be related to particle size and the ability to pass into the distal airway. The formulation of the agent greatly plays a role in the particle size. With the banning of chloroflourocarbons (CFCs), newly developed hydroflouroalkanes (HFAs) were developed with some companies altering the particle sizes. Metered dose inhalers (MDIs) were similarly altered to decrease particle size with solution MDIs resulting in smaller more aerosolized particles with inhalation. Overall, it appears that dry powder inhaler (DPI) steroids, suspension CFCs, and suspension HFA MDI inhalers have greater particle sizes than solution HFA MDIs **(Table 1)**.[14] The smaller particle size of solution HFA MDIs has increased lung deposition from 20% to greater than 50%. Many studies have confirmed greater lung deposition in smaller particle formulations in addition to lower oropharyngeal and laryngeal deposition, lessening oral candidiasis and dysphonia side effects associated with ICSs.[15]

A 2013 Cochrane review of 6 studies comparing ciclesonide, which is a new small-particle ICS, to other ICSs in children did not demonstrate superior benefit over other fluticasones or budesonide.[16] The lung deposition of combination therapy HFA fluticasone/salmeterol compared with HFA beclomethasone was investigated by Leach and colleagues.[17] The smaller-particle HFA beclomethasone (0.7 μm) was found to have 58% of its particles deposited into the lungs compared with 16% of HFA fluticasone/salmeterol (2.7 μm) implying greater potential efficacy and fewer dosing intervals.

The effectiveness of ICS therapy has also been linked to patient compliance factors. ICSs are prescribed at daily dosing intervals of once or twice daily, with most patients achieving control at low doses. Some patients with asthma take ICSs only during periods of asthma exacerbations or worsening symptoms. A 2013 study looking at the outcomes of intermittent versus daily ICS use in children and adults found no significant difference in overall asthma attacks.[18] However, increased frequency of rescue inhaler use, fewer symptom-free days, and decreased lung function were observed in those taking the medication only intermittently. Furthermore, it has been demonstrated that patients who stop routine use of ICSs have an increased risk of asthma exacerbation with decreased FEV1, decreased peak flow, and increased asthma symptom scores.[19]

Steroid therapy and the effects on growth rate has been a concern particularly in the pediatric population with asthma. At lower doses, there is minimal systemic absorption of ICSs. Higher doses of ICSs have been shown to retard growth in children and result in adrenal suppression. Other side effects with long-term use at high doses include osteoporosis, dermal thinning, periodontal disease, cataracts, and glaucoma.

Oral Corticosteroids

Oral corticosteroids are indicated for patients with severe persistent asthma despite management with high-dose ICSs or LABA. Oral corticosteroids are also used in cases of asthma exacerbations. The mechanism of action is similar to that outlined

Table 1		
Lung deposition and particle size comparison of steroid inhalers		
Inhaled Steroid	MMAD (μm)	Lung Deposition Value (%)
Fluticasone DPI	~4.0	15
Triamcinolone	4.5	14
CFC-flunisolide	3.8	19
CFC-beclomethasone	3.5	8
CFC-fluticasone	2.6	13
HFA-flunisolide solution	1.2	68
HFA-beclomethasone solution	1.1	56
HFA-ciclesonide solution	1.0	52

Abbreviations: CFC, chlorofluorocarbon; DPI, dry powder inhaler; HFA, hydrofluoroalkane; MMAD, median mass aerodynamic diameter.
From Leach C, Colice GL, Luskin AC. Particle size of inhaled corticosteroids: does it matter? J Allergy Clin Immunol 2009;124(Suppl 6):S88–93; with permission.

with ICSs; however, greater risk of systemic adverse side effects are observed with chronic use of oral corticosteroids.

LEUKOTRIENE MODIFIERS

LTRAs are recommended as a sole or adjunct therapy for patients with mild persistent asthma to decrease airway edema, bronchoconstriction, and inflammation. The mechanism of action of these agents is through the eicosanoid pathway by inhibiting the binding of cysteinyl leukotrienes (LTC4, LTD4, LTE4) from binding to cysteinyl receptors located on inflammatory cells and airway smooth muscle. Montelukast binds selectively to the cystLT1 receptor predominantly affecting the binding of LTD4. Zafirkulast selectively and competitively binds to receptors for LTD4 and LTE4 influencing both early and late phase hypersensitivity responses. Zileuton is an inhibitor of 5-lipoxygenase, thus affecting the production of LTB4, LTC4, LTD4, and LTE4. Current use of this medication is for ages 12 and older and per NAEPP recommendation is not a preferred agent due to limited studies and need to monitor liver function.

A 2012 Cochrane review comparing leukotriene modifiers to ICS suggested that antileukotrienes may have fewer adverse side effects, but as a monotherapy were not as effective as ICSs.[20]

THEOPHYLLINE

Theophylline is a methylxanthine, indicated as a sole agent for mild persistent asthma or as an adjunct therapy in more severe persistent patients with asthma with ICS. Its mechanism of action is through nonselective phosphodiesterase inhibition. Theophylline serves as a bronchodilator that can be used as an alternative to LABA. The serum concentration of theophylline must be monitored because of the narrow therapeutic index, variable hepatic clearance, and subsequent risk of cardiac arrhythmias and seizures. Diet, cardiac disease, liver disease, tobacco use, and medications that influence the cytochrome P450 system can modify the half-life of theophylline.

MAST CELL STABILIZERS

Mast cell stabilizers, such as inhaled cromolyn sodium, are primarily recommended as an alternative therapy to SABAs and LTRAs for exercise-induced bronchospasm or patients with mild persistent asthma. These agents prevent degranulation of mast cells by preventing calcium uptake into the cell, thereby playing a role in acute and late-phase responses. Netzer and colleagues,[21] after review of the literature, suggested the potential role of cromolyn sodium in the management of asthma, despite current guidelines, because of its potent anti-inflammatory effects, few side effects, and acceptable dosing making it a viable initial option for the control of asthma.

ANTI–IMMUNOGLOBULIN E THERAPY

Omalizumab is a monoclonal anti–immunoglobulin E (anti-IgE) antibody administered as a subcutaneous injection indicated for patients with severe persistent asthma who are 12 years or older and who have demonstrated underlying IgE-mediated allergies. Omalizumab selectively binds to the high-affinity IgE receptor region on IgE preventing its binding to IgE surface receptors on cells ultimately forming immune complexes that decrease available free IgE. It has also been shown to downregulate the expression of high-affinity receptors on inflammatory cells.[22] By inhibiting IgE from binding to its receptors leads to inhibition of the allergic response through inhibition of degranulation of mast cells and basophils, decreased response to antigen challenges, and a decrease in IgE-switching cytokines interleukin (IL)-4 and IL-13. The immune complexes formed by omalizumab can also bind allergens resulting in neutralization of antigen stimulus.

Reported side effects of omalizumab have included the risk of anaphylaxis of about 0.09% based on the Omalizumab Joint Task Force investigations.[22]

Most of these reactions were within the first 2 to 3 hours of the initial 3 injections and within 30 minutes after later injections. All patients responded to anaphylaxis treatment without any fatalities. Other reports of adverse effects include the risk of malignancy; however, it has been concluded that there is no increased risk of malignancy. Other reported adverse reactions include skin reactions, upper respiratory infection, and sinusitis.

In patients with severe allergic asthma uncontrolled with ICS and LABAs, evidence has shown an increased benefit when adding omalizumab to the treatment regimen. Hanania and colleagues,[23] in a randomized, double-blind placebo-controlled trial showed in a 48-week study of patients with uncontrolled allergic asthma that omalizumab reduced asthma exacerbations, albuterol rescue inhaler use, and overall quality of life.

SPECIFIC IMMUNOTHERAPY

Specific immunotherapy (SIT) has been shown to be effective as an adjunctive treatment in managing asthma. Data have consistently shown that immunotherapy decreases medication usage, and reduces asthma symptoms and airway hyperresponsiveness. A recent 2013 review of randomized control trials found that single-allergen subcutaneous immunotherapy (SCIT) improved asthma symptoms and medication usage compared with placebo and pharmacotherapy, suggesting that there may not be a role for multiple allergen immunotherapy.[24] The review also included sublingual immunotherapy (SLIT), which demonstrated an even stronger improvement in asthma symptoms compared with placebo, with most studies evaluating dust mite single-allergen therapy. Randomized controlled trials comparing the efficacy of SCIT to SLIT in improving asthma symptoms are limited and variable. Overall, SIT has been shown to be safe, with most reactions being minor local reactions. In comparison, SLIT appears to have a better safety profile than SCIT. The disadvantages of this line of therapy include the cost, time commitment, and the potential for initial worsening in asthma symptoms.

FUTURE THERAPY

The allergic reaction represents a TH2-dominant response and has been demonstrated in allergic asthma. One novel therapy serves to shift the response to a TH1-mediated protective response by injecting a Toll-like receptor 9 agonist, QbG10. Beeh and colleagues,[25] in a double-blind randomized trial, investigated its role in controlling mild to moderate persistent allergic asthma over a 12-week period compared with placebo. At the completion of the study, two-thirds of QbG10 patients had well-controlled asthma compared with one-third in the placebo group. Additionally, the FEV1 clinically worsened in the placebo group. Side effects to injections were mainly local skin reactions. Other anti-inflammatory therapies with promising results are targeting cytokines, such as IL-4 receptors, IL-5 monoclonal antibody (mepolizumab), anti-IL-9, resiquimod targeting IL-12, anti-IL-13, and MMP-12–specific inhibitor.[26–29]

Steroid resistance has been described in patients with severe persistent asthma and in patients with asthma who smoke. Several molecular mechanisms for steroid resistance have been identified, including a genetic susceptibility or familial glucocorticoid resistance. Other mechanisms include glucocorticoid receptor (GR) modifications, increased GR-beta expression, increased proinflammatory transcription factors, immune mechanisms, and defective histone acetylation via histone deacetylase (HDAC2). Delineation of these mechanisms has become a target for alternative therapies in patients with steroid-resistant asthma and patients with COPD.[30] Oral roflumilast is a phosphodiesterase-4 inhibitor that is the first anti-inflammatory marketed for COPD. P38MAPK inhibitors are being developed to suppress inflammation in patients with asthma and patients with COPD by affecting the mitogen-activated protein kinase (MAPK) pathways normally inhibited by steroids. Reversing steroid resistance by increasing HDAC2 expression, thereby lessening oxidative stress, has also been demonstrated in patients with COPD. Several drugs increase HDAC2, including theophylline and nortriptyline. LABAs also appear to reverse steroid resistance via multiple mechanisms.

Some investigations aim to provide a more personalized approach to asthma management. One such study investigated children carrying the β2- adrenoreceptor gene Arg 16 polymorphism. Patients with this gene appeared to respond better to ICS and LTRA over ICS/LABA suggesting a role for genotyping patients with asthma.[31] Asthmatic patients expressing certain polymorphisms for nitric oxide synthase enzyme appear to have greater response to ICS/LABA combination therapy.[32]

SUMMARY

The NAEPP has provided evidence-based guidelines for the management of asthma. These guidelines allow for standardization of therapy in an effort to improve asthma outcomes. In patients with persistent asthma symptoms, ICS alone or in combination with LABAs have shown to significantly reduce asthma symptoms. Unfortunately, some patients remain refractory to this treatment, requiring more advanced therapy, such as anti-IgE therapy. Other novel therapies are being investigated to treat these refractory patients targeting steroid resistance, genetic, and anti-inflammatory mechanisms.

REFERENCES

1. National Asthma Education and Prevention Program. Expert panel report 3: guidelines for the diagnosis and management of asthma. NIH Publication; 2007. 07–4051.

2. Cazzola M, Page CP, Rogliani P, et al. β2-agonist therapy in lung disease. Am J Respir Crit Care Med 2013;187(7):690–6.
3. Castle W, Fuller R, Hall J, et al. Serevent nationwide surveillance study: comparison of salmeterol with salbutamol in asthmatic patients who require regular bronchodilator treatment. BMJ 1993;306:1034–7.
4. Nelson HS, Weiss ST, Bleecker ER, et al. The salmeterol multicenter asthma research trial: a comparison of usual pharmacotherapy for asthma or usual pharmacotherapy plus salmeterol. Chest 2006;129:15–26.
5. Mann M, Chowdhury B, Sullivan E, et al. Serious asthma exacerbations in asthmatics treated with high-dose formoterol. Chest 2003;124:70–4.
6. Chowdhury BA, Dal Pan G. The FDA and safe use of long acting beta agonists in the treatment of asthma. N Engl J Med 2010;362:1169–71.
7. Lasserson TJ, Ferrara G, Casali L. Combination fluticasone and salmeterol versus fixed dose combination budesonide and formoterol for chronic asthma in adults and children. Cochrane Database Syst Rev 2011;(12):CD004106.
8. Aalbers R, Brusselle G, McIver T, et al. Onset of bronchodilation with fluticasone/formoterol combination versus fluticasone/sameterol in an open-label, randomized study. Adv Ther 2012;29(11):958–69.
9. Hojo M, Mizutani T, Iikura M, et al. Asthma control can be maintained after fixed-dose, budesonide/formoterol combination inhaler therapy is stepped down from medium to low dose. Allergol Int 2013;62:91–8.
10. Kerstjens HA, Engel M, Dahl R, et al. Tiotropium in asthma poorly controlled with standard combination therapy. N Engl J Med 2012;367:1198–207.
11. Townley RG, Suliaman F. The mechanism of corticosteroids in treating asthma. Ann Allergy 1987;58(1):1–6.
12. Jang A. Steroid response in refractory asthmatics. Korean J Intern Med 2012;27: 143–8.
13. Lawrence M, Wolfe J, Webb DR, et al. Efficacy of inhaled fluticasone propionate in asthma results from topical and not from systemic activity. Am J Respir Crit Care Med 1997;156:744–51.
14. Leach C, Colice GL, Luskin AC. Particle size of inhaled corticosteroids: does it matter? J Allergy Clin Immunol 2009;124(Suppl 6):S88–93.
15. van den Berge M, ten Hacken NH, van der Wiel E, et al. Treatment of the bronchial tree from beginning to end: targeting small airway inflammation in asthma. Allergy 2013;68:16–26.
16. Kramer S, Rottier BL, Scholten RJ, et al. Ciclesonide versus other inhaled corticosteroids for chronic asthma in children. Cochrane Database Syst Rev 2013;(2):CD010352.
17. Leach CL, Kuehl PJ, Ramesh C, et al. Characterization of respiratory deposition of fluticasone-salmeterol hydrofluoroalkane-134a and hydroflouroalkane-134a beclomethasone in asthmatic patients. Ann Allergy Asthma Immunol 2012;108: 135–200.
18. Chauhan BF, Chartrand C, Ducharme FM. Intermittent versus daily inhaled corticosteroids for persistent asthma in children and adults. Cochrane Database Syst Rev 2013;(2):CD009611.
19. Rank MA, Hagan JB, Park MA, et al. The risk of asthma exacerbation after stopping low-dose inhaled corticosteroids: a systematic review and meta-analysis of randomized control trials. J Allergy Clin Immunol 2013;131:724–9.
20. Chauhan BF, Ducharme FM. Anti-leukotriene agents compared to inhaled corticosteroids in the management of recurrent and/or chronic asthma in adults and children. Cochrane Database Syst Rev 2012;(5):CD002314.

21. Netzer NC, Küpper T, Voss HW, et al. The actual role of sodium cromoglycate in the treatment of asthma—a critical review. Sleep Breath 2012;16:1027–32.

22. Pelaia G, Gallelli L, Renda T, et al. Update on optimal use of omalizumab in management of asthma. J Asthma Allergy 2011;4:49–59.

23. Hanania NA, Alpan O, Hamilos DL, et al. Omalizumab in severe allergic asthma inadequately controlled with standard therapy: a randomized trial. Ann Intern Med 2011;154(9):573–82.

24. Kim JM, Lin SY, Suarez-Cuervo C, et al. Allergen-specific immunotherapy for pediatric asthma and rhinoconjunctivitis: a systematic review. Pediatrics 2013;131: 1155–67.

25. Beeh K, Kanniess F, Wagner F, et al. The novel TLR-9 agonist QbG10 shows clinical efficacy in persistent allergic asthma. J Allergy Clin Immunol 2013;131: 866–74.

26. Chang C. Asthma in children and adolescents: a comprehensive approach to diagnosis and management. Clin Rev Allergy Immunol 2012;43:98–137.

27. Hansbro PM, Scott GV, Essilfie A, et al. Th2 cytokine antagonists: potential treatments for severe asthma. Expert Opin Investig Drugs 2013;22(1):49–69.

28. Ingram JL, Krat M. IL-13 in asthma and allergic disease: asthma phenotypes and targeted therapies. J Allergy Clin Immunol 2012;130:829–42.

29. Pavord ID, Korn S, Howarth P, et al. Mepolizumab for severe eosinophilic asthma (DREAM): a multicentre, double-blind, placebo controlled trial. Lancet 2012;380: 651–9.

30. Barnes PJ. Corticosteroid resistance in patients with asthma and chronic obstructive pulmonary disease. J Allergy Clin Immunol 2013;131:636–45.

31. Lipworth BJ, Basu K, Donald HP, et al. Tailored second line therapy in asthmatic children with the Arg 16 genotype. Clin Sci (Lond) 2013;124:521–8.

32. Iordanidou M, Paraskakis E, Tavridou A, et al. G894T polymorphism of eNOS gene is a predictor of response t combination of inhaled corticosteroids with long-lasting β2- agonist in asthmatic children. Pharmacogenomics 2012;13(12): 1363–72.

Stepwise Treatment of Asthma

John A. Fornadley, MD

KEYWORDS

- Bronchospasm • Intermittent bronchospasm • Persistent bronchospasm

KEY POINTS

- Asthma management is based on severity of disease.
- Overmedication or undermedication of asthma is a concern.
- Uncontrolled asthma may lead to irreversible lung disease.

Step therapy for treatment of asthma has proven a successful means of guiding practitioners through marked changes in management strategy and of gaining better control over this difficult disease process.

In the middle to late twentieth century, asthma therapy was not providing satisfactory control of the disease. Physician visits, self-reported reactive airway disease prevalence, and deaths due to asthma increased between 1960 and 1990.[1–4] Even more troubling was that a percentage of the deaths were attributed to the bronchodilator therapy, specifically exacerbations of disease related to long-acting beta2-agonist (LABA) use. Even without these concerns, bronchodilator therapy did not seem to be the definitive therapy to manage asthma.

Scientific work in the 1960s included the discovery of IgE and a better delineation of the role of inflammation in reversible airway disease.[5] In combination with recently developed inhaled corticosteroids, this provided a better understanding of the disease as well as a pathway that could make a substantial positive impact on the quality of life for a patient with asthma.

Several challenges surrounded the acceptance of this radical algorithm change. The first was the need to educate and change practice patterns of the wide range of practitioners treating asthma, which required informing them and gaining their acceptance of the strategy. Unlike a new medication or adjunctive therapy, the concept of inflammation-based therapy for asthma represented a marked philosophic change. Because physicians tend to gather their continuing education from the medical journals and societies related to their specific field, there was a need to reach out to several disparate societies and journals to get information to the practitioners regarding changes in the therapy of asthma.

Department of Surgery, Penn State University, 500 University Drive, Hershey, PA 17036, USA
E-mail address: entshop@aol.com

Otolaryngol Clin N Am 47 (2014) 65–75
http://dx.doi.org/10.1016/j.otc.2013.09.014
0030-6665/14/$ – see front matter © 2014 Elsevier Inc. All rights reserved.

Asthma therapy is also complicated by the variability of the disease from life-threatening exacerbations to a completely normal quality of life between episodes. This disease process does not lend itself to simply starting a medication and continuing it routinely for years, as in the case of hypertension or types of cardiac disease. There is a legitimate concern among physicians and patients about overmedication or undermedication of asthma. Without guidelines, it was unclear when it would be most appropriate to start medications. Unfortunately, with the medications involved, there were side effect profiles that made overuse undesirable. Steroid therapy, which represented a critical new role in asthma care, is known to have side effects that include growth retardation, decreased immunocompetence, and multiple system-based complications. All branches of medicine recognize a strong desire to limit steroid use, which complicates acceptance of the new regimen. In asthma, these limitations must be balanced against the risk of progression of disease and the inability to stabilize the airway by other means.

Beta agonists have a somewhat diminished but still vital role in the more modern therapy approach. These agents also suffer from reported complications, including electrolyte disorders, cardiac dysrhythmias, and sudden death.[2,4]

This change in asthma management occurred at a time when clinical practice guidelines were less well understood and certainly less trusted. Current data on the value of evidence-based guidelines were obviously not available and the physicians of the time were concerned that guidelines were intended to restrict testing and control medical practices for the benefit of third-party payers.

It was in this medical environment that the National Asthma Education and Prevention Program (NAEPP), under the auspices of the National Heart, Lung, and Blood Institute, performed a thorough literature review and created a guideline pathway for asthma that was published in 1991.[6] The guidelines have been revised in 1997, 2002, and most recently in 2007. The guideline divided asthma into categories of intermittent or persistent, with the latter category being subdivided into mild, moderate, or severe. This categorization then provided the clinician with a step therapy based on the severity of the asthma. These pathways have largely succeeded in changing the way asthma is managed, starting in the last decade of the twentieth century. The intervening time has allowed statistical analysis to identify actual improvement in asthma management as measured by fewer emergency visits and deaths.

From 1991 to 2006, progress in the field, new medications, and updated data resulted in the need for changes to the asthma management algorithm. The stepwise approach has grown necessarily more complicated, but the overall principles remain. The guideline continues to provide some rigidity but allows physician judgment and insight. In the current version, the guidelines include patient education and some patient responsibilities. Although some of the elegant simplicity of the 1991 algorithm is lost, the present update allows better active consideration of allergic components of the disease. In addition, there are more options for effectively allowing medication use to step up when needed and step down when possible.

The now-familiar four categories of asthma remain unchanged. The step approach for asthma therapy has increased these to six steps. The care recommendations are stratified for patient ages of 0 to 4 years, 5 to 11 years, and 12-plus years to allow for better treatment of pediatric medication variances.

The initial step, as before, is the diagnosis of asthma. The goal is to identify asthma, evaluate and exclude other diagnoses, and determine the severity of the disease. Patient history, spirometry (in patients older than 5 years), and the exclusion of other diagnoses is important in arriving at the correct diagnosis. The severity of the disease is important in determining how to initiate therapy. The control aspect of disease is vital in monitoring and controlling therapy. Severity is defined as the intrinsic intensity of the disease process. This parameter is important for the initiation of therapy (**Table 1**).

The initial assessment is the first and arguably the most critical step, because it has a role in both diagnosis and the direction of initial therapy. The steps of the initial assessment are illustrated in **Table 1**. Note that the diagnosis includes a history of symptoms and types of precipitating factors, not only spirometry. Spirometry is nevertheless required in patients 5 years and older. These historical data combined with the results of spirometry assist the clinician in making the diagnosis of asthma and provides for patient stratification into a defined level of asthma severity.

Because this clinical information is vital to the correct categorization of the patient's level of asthma, the clinician should be familiar with **Table 1** when taking the asthma history. In addition to categorization into intermittent versus persistent, and as mild, moderate, or severe, the patients are also grouped according to age. Based on the level of findings, the clinician is directed to a subsequent algorithm that indicates the recommended medical therapeutic selection (**Table 2**).

CRITICAL CHANGES IN THE THIRD REVISION

The updated guidelines reflect a identified need to monitor the control of asthma. Whereas the initial evaluation of the patient with asthma is to determine at which step to initiate therapy, the reassessments are geared to determine the control of therapy and the need to adjust medications. The evaluation with ongoing therapy is to assess whether the patient's quality of life has improved by the control of symptoms as outlined in the written physician-patient plan. The evaluation should allow a determination of whether medication use should increase (step up) or decrease (step down). This permits the best quality of life with minimal medication use.

In addition to the medication therapy, the guidelines make education a central component to therapy. This includes assuring that the patient understands self-monitoring of asthma control and can identify signs of acute exacerbation or generalized worsening of disease. Education also encompasses the correct way of physically taking the medications and the decision process for the use of rescue medications. Finally, education extends to the lifestyle changes vital to minimizing asthmatic episodes.

Emphasis is placed on a written asthma plan, which is to be created individually for the patient and reviewed regularly between the patient and physician.

Allergic disease also receives recognition and therapeutic recommendations in the 2007 version of the guidelines.[7] The second expert panel acknowledged the inflammatory component of asthma and the genetic disposition to atopic disease as a major factor. However, the most recent guideline takes the singular step of advocating allergy immunotherapy in cases where a clear connection exists "between symptoms and exposure to an allergen to which the patient is sensitive."[8] This is an important comment for several reasons. Patients with asthma have a higher risk of adverse response to immunotherapy. There have been questions in the literature about whether allergy immunotherapy is sufficiently helpful in the control of asthma to make it worth the risks of adverse reaction. The inclusion of immunotherapy by the expert panel seems to address these concerns, approving the use of immunotherapy in mild to moderate persistent disease, at least in cases in which a direct link to asthma can be appreciated.[9]

Recommendations that are more specific are possible when patients are grouped into 0 to 4 year olds and 5 to 11 year olds. The latter group was represented as a portion of the adult recommendations in earlier versions of the expert panel recommendations.

Table 1
Initial visit: classifying asthma severity and initiating therapy (in patients who are not currently taking long-term control medications)

| Components of Severity | | Intermittent | | | Persistent | | | | | | | | | |
| | | | | | Mild | | | Moderate | | | Severe | | | |
		Ages 0–4 y	Ages 5–11 y	Ages ≥12 y	Ages 0–4 y	Ages 5–11 y	Ages ≥12 y	Ages 0–4 y	Ages 5–11 y	Ages ≥12 y	Ages 0–4 y	Ages 5–11 y	Ages ≥12 y
Impairment	Symptoms		≤2 d/wk			>2 d/wk but not daily			Daily			Throughout the day	
	Nighttime awakenings	0	≤2x/mo		1–2x/mo	3–4x/mo		3–4x/mo	>1x/wk but not nightly		>1x/wk	Several times per day	Often 7x/wk
	SABA use for symptom control (not to prevent EIB)		≤2 d/wk		>2 d/wk but not daily	>2 d/wk but not daily and not more than once on any day		Daily			Several times per day	
	Interference with normal activity	None			Minor limitation			Some limitation			Extremely limited	
	Lung function		Normal FEV₁ between exacerbations	Normal FEV₁ between exacerbations		Minor limitation			Some limitation			Extremely limited	
	↓ FEV₁ (% predicted)	Not applicable	>80%	>80%	Not applicable	>80%	>80%	Not applicable	60%–80%	60%–80%	Not applicable	<60%	<60%
	↓ FEV₁/FVC		>85%	Normal[a]		>80%	Normal[a]		75%–80%	75%–80%		<75%	<75%
Risk	Asthma exacerbations requiring oral systemic corticosteroids[b]	0–1/y	0–1/y	0–1/y	≥2 exacerb. in 6 mo, or wheezing ≥4x per y lasting >1d AND risk factors for persistent asthma	≥2/y	≥2/y					Reduced 5%[a]	Reduced >5%[a]

Consider severity and interval since last asthma exacerbation. Frequency and severity may fluctuate over time for patients in any severity category.
Relative annual risk of exacerbations may be related to FEV₁.

Generally, more frequent and intense events indicate greater severity.

Recommended Step for Initiating Therapy (See "Stepwise Approach for Managing Asthma Long Term")	Step 1			Step 2			Step 3	Step 3 medium-dose ICS option	Step 3 medium-dose ICS option	Step 3	Step 3 medium-dose ICS option or Step 4	Step 4 or 5

The stepwise approach is meant to help, not replace, the clinical decisionmaking needed to meet individual patient needs.

In 2–6 wk, depending on severity, assess level of asthma control achieved and adjust therapy as needed.

Consider short course of oral systemic corticosteroids.

For children 0–4 y old, if no clear benefit is observed in 4–6 wk, consider adjusting therapy or alternate diagnoses.

Level of severity (columns 2–5) is determined by events listed in column 1 for both impairment (frequency and intensity of symptoms and functional limitations) and risk (of exacerbations). Assess impairment by patient's or caregiver's recall of events during the previous 2 to 4 weeks; assess risk over the last year. Recommendations for initiating therapy based on level of severity are presented in the last row.

Abbreviations: EIB, exercise-induced bronchospasm; FEV$_1$, forced expiratory volume in 1 second; FVC, forced vital capacity; ICS, inhaled corticosteroid; SABA, short-acting beta2-agonist.

[a] Normal FEV$_1$/FVC by age: 8–19 y, 85%; 20–39 y, 80%; 40–59 y, 75%; 60–80 y, 70%.

[b] Data are insufficient to link frequencies of exacerbations with different levels of asthma severity. Generally, more frequent and intense exacerbations (eg, requiring urgent care, hospital or intensive care admission, and/or oral corticosteroids) indicate greater underlying disease severity. For treatment purposes, patients with ≥2 exacerbations may be considered to have persistent asthma, even in the absence of impairment levels consistent with persistent asthma.

From National Heart, Lung, and Blood Institute. Asthma care quick reference. Available at: http://www.nhlbi.nih.gov/guidelines/asthma/asthma_qrg.pdf. Accessed September 17, 2013.

Table 2
Stepwise approach for managing asthma long-term

		STEP 1	STEP 2	STEP 3	STEP 4	STEP 5	STEP 6

ASSESS CONTROL:

STEP UP IF NEEDED (first, check medication adherence, inhaler technique, environmental control, and comorbidities)

STEP DOWN IF POSSIBLE (and asthma is well controlled for at least 3 mo)

At each step: Patient education, environmental control, and management of comorbidities

0–4 y of age

	STEP 1	STEP 2	STEP 3	STEP 4	STEP 5	STEP 6
	Intermittent Asthma	Persistent Asthma: Daily Medication — Consult with asthma specialist if step 3 care or higher is required. Consider consultation at step 2.				
Preferred Treatment[a]	SABA as needed	low-dose ICS	medium-dose ICS	medium-dose ICS + either LABA or montelukast	high-dose ICS + either LABA or montelukast	high-dose ICS + either LABA or montelukast + oral corticosteroids
Alternative Treatment[a,b]		cromolyn or montelukast				

If clear benefit is not observed in 4–6 wk, and medication technique and adherence are satisfactory, consider adjusting therapy or alternate diagnoses.

Quick-Relief Medication	• SABA as needed for symptoms; intensity of treatment depends on severity of symptoms. • With viral respiratory symptoms: SABA every 4–6 h up to 24 h (longer with physician consult). Consider short course of oral systemic corticosteroids if asthma exacerbation is severe or patient has history of severe exacerbations. • Caution: Frequent use of SABA may indicate the need to step up treatment.

5–11 y of age

	STEP 1	STEP 2	STEP 3	STEP 4	STEP 5	STEP 6
	Intermittent Asthma	Persistent Asthma: Daily Medication — Consult with asthma specialist if step 4 care or higher is required. Consider consultation at step 3.				
Preferred Treatment[a]	SABA as needed	low-dose ICS	low-dose ICS + either LABA, LTRA, or theophylline[b]	medium-dose ICS + LABA	high-dose ICS + LABA	high-dose ICS + LABA + oral corticosteroids
Alternative Treatment[a,b]		cromolyn, LTRA, or theophylline[c]	OR medium-dose ICS	medium-dose ICS + either LTRA or theophylline[c]	high-dose ICS + either LTRA or theophylline[c]	high-dose ICS + either LTRA or theophylline[c] + oral corticosteroids

Consider subcutaneous allergen immunotherapy for patients who have persistent, allergic asthma.

Quick-Relief Medication	• SABA as needed for symptoms. The intensity of treatment depends on severity of symptoms: up to 3 treatments every 20 min as needed. Short course of oral systemic corticosteroids may be needed. • Caution: Increasing use of SABA or use >2 d/wk for symptom relief (not to prevent EIB) generally indicates inadequate control and the need to step up treatment.

≥12 y of age

	STEP 1	STEP 2	STEP 3	STEP 4	STEP 5	STEP 6
	Intermittent Asthma	Persistent Asthma: Daily Medication — Consult with asthma specialist if step 4 care or higher is required. Consider consultation at step 3.				
Preferred Treatment[a]	SABA as needed	low-dose ICS	low-dose ICS + LABA OR medium-dose ICS	medium-dose ICS + LABA	high-dose ICS + LABA AND consider omalizumab for patients who have allergies[e]	high-dose ICS + LABA + oral corticosteroid[f] AND consider omalizumab for patients who have allergies[e]
Alternative Treatment[a,b]		cromolyn, LTRA, or theophylline[c]	low-dose ICS + either LTRA, theophylline,[c] or zileuton[d]	medium-dose ICS + either LTRA, theophylline,[c] or zileuton[d]		

Consider subcutaneous allergen immunotherapy for patients who have persistent, allergic asthma.

Quick-Relief Medication	• SABA as needed for symptoms. The intensity of treatment depends on severity of symptoms: up to 3 treatments every 20 min as needed. Short course of oral systemic corticosteroids may be needed. • Caution: Use of SABA >2 d/wk for symptom relief (not to prevent EIB) generally indicates inadequate control and the need to step up treatment.

The stepwise approach tailors the selection of medication to the level of asthma severity or asthma control. The stepwise approach is meant to help, not replace, the clinical decision making needed to meet individual patient needs.

Abbreviations: EIB, exercise-induced bronchospasm; ICS, inhaled corticosteroid; LTRA, leukotriene receptor antagonist; SABA, short-acting beta2-agonist (inhaled).

[a] Treatment options are listed in alphabetical order, if more than one.

[b] If alternative treatment is used and response is inadequate, discontinue and use preferred treatment before stepping up.

[c] Theophylline is a less desirable alternative because of the need to monitor serum concentration levels. Based on evidence for dust mites, animal dander, and pollen; evidence is weak or lacking for molds and cockroaches. Evidence is strongest for immunotherapy with single allergens. The role of allergy in asthma is greater in children than in adults.

[d] Zileuton is less desirable because of limited studies as adjunctive therapy and the need to monitor liver function.

[e] Clinicians who administer immunotherapy or omalizumab should be prepared to treat anaphylaxis that may occur.

[f] Before oral corticosteroids are introduced, a trial of high-dose ICS + LABA + either LTRA, theophylline, or zileuton, may be considered, although this approach has not been studied in clinical trials.

From National Heart, Lung, and Blood Institute. Asthma care quick reference. Available at: http://www.nhlbi.nih.gov/guidelines/asthma/asthma_qrg.pdf. Accessed September 17, 2013.

STEPPING THROUGH THE PROCESS OF STEPWISE CARE
The Asthma Diagnosis

The frequency of symptoms, nighttime awakenings, and use of short-acting beta2-agonists (SABA) combined with spirometry data are the first level used to categorize the severity of asthma. Next it is categorized by intermittent versus persistent. The persistent category is subdivided into mild-moderate or severe. The diagnosis of severity is based on these four categories (see **Table 1**).

Once asthma severity is categorized, the clinician has guidelines to choose from six levels of therapy. Having more levels of therapy than categories of severity allows a different starting point for pediatric and adult patients. It also provides more flexibility in stepping up and down the regimen for patients who require only subtle changes in therapy. Alternative therapies are noted as appropriate (see **Table 2**).

In all age groups, intermittent asthma is managed with step 1 therapy. This primary level therapy is the use of a SABA on an as-needed basis. There is no alternative treatment needed or appropriate at this level.

Mild persistent asthma is the second category. At this level, alternative therapies can be considered. Essentially, the primary or recommended therapy is low-dose inhaled corticosteroids. An alternative therapy includes cromolyn, leukotriene receptor antagonists, or (5 years and older) theophylline. This provides the option to withhold inhaled corticosteroids if there is a strong patient or parental concern. Although these two alternative therapies are considered equivalent for the management of mild intermittent asthma, studies indicate that inhaled corticosteroids may better prevent inflammation, and decrease risk of exacerbation and subsequent airway remodeling. Step 2 is also the first level at which subcutaneous allergen immunotherapy should be considered for patients with allergic disease that clearly relates to asthma exacerbations. The data are considered stronger for allergy exacerbating asthma in children and the best evidence seems to support allergy against dust mites, animal dander, and pollen.[9]

Moderate persistent asthma is initially treated with step 3 therapy. This involves the use of low-dose inhaled corticosteroids plus an LABA or the use of medium-dose inhaled corticosteroids alone. An alternative for adults is to avoid the LABA by substituting leukotriene receptor antagonists or theophylline. A similar option exists for children 5 to 11 years old. The youngest children requiring step 3 therapy are managed using medium-dose inhaled corticosteroids alone.

Severe persistent asthma is managed in adults using medium dose inhaled corticosteroids and LABA. An alternative of medium dose inhaled corticosteroids with theophylline or a leukotriene receptor antagonist is also an option. Some adults may exhibit such a severe level of asthma that they require initiation with therapy above step 4 care. Step 5 is high-dose inhaled corticosteroids, combined with LABA, with consideration given to the use of oral steroids. Once step 5 or step 6 is reached, allergy immunotherapy is no longer a recommendation. At this level of asthma, the risk of triggering a significant exacerbation outweighs the benefits of allergy immunotherapy. At this level of severity in the allergic population, omalizumab may be used as replacement for allergy immunotherapy for step 5 and 6 care.[10]

Step 6 is not used as a starting level, but has been added to the guidelines to provide a rational increased level of care for patients experiencing incomplete control on follow-up visits. Step 6 includes oral corticosteroids in all age groups in addition to high-dose inhaled corticosteroids. LABA is recommended all age groups at level 6.

As previously noted, patient's should leave the initial visit with medical therapy based on the severity of the disease. They should receive education about the disease

Table 3
Follow-up visits: assessing asthma control and adjusting therapy

Components of Control	Well Controlled — Ages 0-4 y	Well Controlled — Ages 5-11 y	Well Controlled — Ages ≥12 y	Not Well Controlled — Ages 0-4 y	Not Well Controlled — Ages 5-11 y	Not Well Controlled — Ages ≥12 y	Very Poorly Controlled — Ages 0-4 y	Very Poorly Controlled — Ages 5-11 y	Very Poorly Controlled — Ages ≥12 y
Impairment									
Symptoms	≤2 d/wk	≤2 d/wk but not more than once on each day	≤2 d/wk	>2 d/wk	>2 d/wk or multiple times on ≤2 d/wk	>2 d/wk	Throughout the day	Throughout the day	Throughout the day
Nighttime awakenings	≤1x/mo	None	≤2x/mo	>1x/mo	≥2x/mo	1-3x/wk	>1x/wk	≥2x/wk	≥4x/wk
Interference with normal activity	None	None	None	Some limitation	Some limitation	Some limitation	Extremely limited	Extremely limited	Extremely limited
SABA use for symptom control (not to prevent EIB)	≤2 d/wk	≤2 d/wk	≤2 d/wk	>2 d/wk	>2 d/wk	>2 d/wk	Several times per day	Several times per day	Several times per day
Lung function — FEV$_1$ (% predicted) or peak flow (% personal/best)	Not applicable	>80%	>80%	Not applicable	60%-80%	60%-80%	Not applicable	<60%	<60%
FEV$_1$/FVC	Not applicable	>80%	Not applicable	Not applicable	75%-80%	Not applicable	Not applicable	<75%	Not applicable
Validated questionnaires[a] — ATAQ	Not applicable	Not applicable	0	Not applicable	Not applicable	1-2	Not applicable	Not applicable	3-4
ACQ	Not applicable	Not applicable	≤0.75[b]	Not applicable	Not applicable	≥1.5	Not applicable	Not applicable	Not applicable
ACT	Not applicable	Not applicable	≥20	Not applicable	Not applicable	16-19	Not applicable	Not applicable	≤15
Risk									
Asthma exacerbations requiring oral systemic corticosteroids[c]	0-1/y	0-1/y	0-1/y	2-3/y	≥2/y	≥2/y	>3/y	≥2/y	≥2/y
			Consider severity and interval since last asthma exacerbation.						
Reduction in lung growth/Progressive loss of lung function	Not applicable	Evaluation requires long-term follow-up care.	Evaluation requires long-term follow-up care.	Not applicable	Evaluation requires long-term follow-up care.	Evaluation requires long-term follow-up care.	Not applicable	Evaluation requires long-term follow-up care.	Evaluation requires long-term follow-up care.
Treatment-related adverse effects				*Medication side effects can vary in intensity from none to very troublesome and worrisome.*					
				The level of intensity does not correlate to specific levels of control but should be considered in the overall assessment of risk.					
Recommended Action for Treatment (See "Stepwise Approach for Managing Asthma Long Term.") The stepwise approach is meant to help, not replace, the clinical decisionmaking needed to meet individual patient needs.	*Maintain current step.* *Regular follow-up every 1-6 mo.* *Consider step down if well controlled for at least 3 mo.*			Step up 1 step *Reevaluate in 2-6 wk to achieve control.* *For children 0-4 y, if no clear benefit observed in 4-6 wk, consider adjusting therapy or alternative diagnoses*	Step up at least 1 step	Step up 1 step *Reevaluate in 2-6 wk to achieve control.*	Consider short course of oral systemic corticosteroids. *Step up 1-2 steps.* *Reevaluate in 2 wk to achieve control.*		
				Before step up in treatment: *Review adherence to medication, inhaler technique, and environmental control. If alternative treatment was used, discontinue and use preferred treatment for that step. For side effects, consider alternative treatment options.*					

Level of control (columns 2–4) is based on the most severe component of impairment (symptoms and functional limitations) or risk (exacerbations). Assess impairment by patient's or caregiver's recall of events listed in column 1 during the previous 2 to 4 weeks and by spirometry and/or peak flow measures. Symptom assessment for longer periods should reflect a global assessment, such as inquiring whether the patient's asthma is better or worse since the last visit. Assess risk by recall of exacerbations during the previous year and since the last visit. Recommendations for adjusting therapy based on level of control are presented in the last row.

Abbreviations: ACQ, Asthma Control Questionnaire; ACT, Asthma Control Test; ATAQ, Asthma Therapy Assessment Questionnaire; EIB, exercise-induced bronchospasm; FEV$_1$, forced expiratory volume in 1 second; FVC, forced vital capacity; SABA, short-acting beta2-agonist.

[a] Minimal important difference: 1.0 for the ATAQ; 0.5 for the ACQ; not determined for the ACT.

[b] ACQ values of 0.76–1.4 are indeterminate regarding well-controlled asthma.

[c] Data are insufficient to link frequencies of exacerbations with different levels of asthma control. Generally, more frequent and intense exacerbations (eg, requiring urgent care, hospital or intensive care admission, and/or oral corticosteroids) indicate poorer asthma control.

From National Heart, Lung, and Blood Institute. Asthma care quick reference. Available at: http://www.nhlbi.nih.gov/guidelines/asthma/asthma_qrg.pdf. Accessed September 17, 2013.

process and ways to monitor their process by means of either symptoms or expiratory flow measures. Lifestyle adjustment information and careful allergy history and testing as appropriate are recommended.

Once therapy has been initiated, follow-up visits are crucial to the step-wise nature of the treatment. Despite all guidelines, the best measure of success in therapy is how the patient progresses. If additional medication is needed, it is important to identify this early in the process and step up the treatment. Similarly, if satisfactory disease control is achieved, reducing medications (step down) will limit the risk of medicine side effects. During the initial phase of asthma therapy, follow-up every 2 to 6 weeks may be necessary. Ongoing asthma management can vary from 1 to 6 months, with spirometry every 1 to 2 years. Follow-up of approximately 3 months is considered most reasonable if the patient is a candidate for decreased therapy. Certainly, if control of asthma is insufficient, visits that are more frequent will be required in order to step up the therapy in a timely fashion.

Although the initial diagnosis is geared mostly to the severity of asthma, follow-up visits are mostly concerned with the level of control achieved on the given step of therapy. **Table 3** defines the asthma has well controlled, not well controlled, or very poorly controlled, based on the most severe component of the patient's impairment. The impairments include nighttime awakenings, interference with normal activity, need for rescue inhaler use (not including exercise-induced bronchospasm).

Objective measures of lung function include forced expiratory volume in 1 second (FEV_1) or peak flow as a percentage of personal best. In children ages 5 to 11 years, the FEV_1 to forced vital capacity (FVC) ratio is a helpful alternative metric.

As an example, adults who wake fewer than two times a month are considered well controlled, whereas those who wake more than four times a week are considered very poorly controlled. Normal activity should be completely free of interference in well-controlled asthma. A patient who has asthma that is not well controlled has some limitation, whereas the patient with poorly controlled asthma is extremely activity-limited. SABA therapy several times a day is an indicator of poor control, whereas more than two days a week is considered not well controlled, and fewer than twice a week defines well-controlled asthma.

At follow-up visits, a patient with well-controlled asthma maintains the same level of medication. The patient is considered for a step down to lower medical regimen if control remains satisfactory for at least 3 months. Patients whose asthma is considered not well controlled or poorly controlled should be evaluated carefully. Before simply adding medications, consideration should be given to the presence of any underlying illness or an unfavorable lifestyle adjustment that has precipitated the unfavorable change. Additionally, the clinician should assess patient compliance to medication regimen and patient understanding and use of satisfactory techniques (particularly for inhalers). Reassessment of allergic disease and the use of environmental controls should be undertaken. If there is no specific deficiency in the present therapy, and the patient is experiencing problems with control, treatment will need to move up at least one step in therapy.

When considering stepping up therapy, two schools of thought have emerged. One is to increase the therapy gradually, one step at a time, while keeping the patient under careful surveillance. This minimizes the additional use of medications and avoids overshooting the appropriate treatment endpoint. The disadvantage of this therapy is that a patient with moderate or severe asthma who is experiencing poor control might experience significant problems, including need for emergency room intervention, before satisfactory control is achieved. The other option is to advance the therapy two or three steps to a near-maximal therapy, often including oral corticosteroids.

The goal is to achieve rapid control of the asthma exacerbation, and then withdraw medical therapy down to a level that allows for a normal lifestyle. The more aggressive approach has reasonable literature support. The belief is that rapid use of additional steroids will decrease airway inflammation and eventually allow patient management at a lower level than if the medications are increased gradually (allowing airway inflammation to be present for a longer time).

SUMMARY

Therapy for asthma has undergone substantial changes in the past three decades, prompted by a better understanding of the role of inflammation in reversible airway disease. Improved therapies and a workable algorithm of step therapy guidelines have provided an improved quality of life for the patient with asthma.

REFERENCES

1. Sly RM. Mortality from asthma, 1979–1984. J Allergy Clin Immunol 1988;82(5 Pt 1): 705–17.
2. Wijesingh M, Weatherall M, Perrin K, et al. International trends in asthma mortality rates in the 5- to 34 year age group: a call for closer surveillance. Chest 2009; 135(4):1045–9.
3. Mannino DM, Homa DM, Pertowski CA, et al. Surveillance for asthma—US 1960–1995. MMWR CDC Surveill Summ 1998;47(SS-1):1–2. Available at: http://www.cdc.gov/mmwr/preview/mmwrhtml/00052262.htm.
4. Barger LW, Vollmer WM, Felt RW, et al. Further investigation into the recent increase in asthma death rates: a review of 41 asthma deaths in Oregon in 1982. Ann Allergy 1988;60(1):31–9.
5. Ishizaka T, Ishizaka K. Molecular basis of reaginic hypersensitivity. Prog Allergy 1975;19:60–121.
6. Guidelines for the diagnosis and management of asthma. National Heart, Lung and Blood Institute. National Asthma Education Program Expert Panel Report. J Allergy Clin Immunol 1991;88(3 pt 2):425–534.
7. National Asthma Education and Prevention Program. 2007 guidelines of the national heart lungs and blood institute; Expert Panel Report 3 (EPR-3): guidelines for the diagnosis and management of asthma-summary report 2007. J Allergy Clin Immunol 2007;120(Suppl 5):S94–138.
8. Hurst DS, Gordon BR, Fornadley JA, et al. Safety of home-based and office allergy immunotherapy: a multicenter prospective study. Otolaryngol Head Neck Surg 1999;121(5):553–61.
9. Lin SY, Erekosima N, Suarez-Cuervo C, et al. Allergen specific immunotherapy for the treatment of allergic rhinoconjunctivitis and/or asthma: comparative effectiveness review 111; ARHQ pub 13 EHC061-EP 2013.
10. Chapman KR, Cartier A, Hébert J, et al. The role of omalizumab in the treatment of severe allergic asthma. Can Respir J 2006;13(Suppl B):1B–9B.

Bronchial Thermoplasty

Jessica Kynyk, MD, Cathy Benninger, RN, MS, CNP,
Karen L. Wood, MD*

KEYWORDS

- Bronchial thermoplasty • Airway smooth muscle • Severe asthma

KEY POINTS

- Bronchial thermoplasty (BT) is a bronchoscopic procedure that involves the direct application of thermal energy to the airways and is performed at 3 separate sessions spaced 3 weeks apart.
- BT leads to the destruction of airway smooth muscle (ASM), because ASM plays an important role in the pathophysiology of asthma.
- The procedure is approved for patients with severe asthma and results in improvement in quality of life and decreased asthma exacerbations.

 A video demonstrating BT accompanies this article at www.oto.theclinics.com

INTRODUCTION

Bronchial thermoplasty (BT) was approved by the Food and Drug Administration (FDA) in April 2010[1] and offers a novel add-on treatment of the management of severe asthma by reducing smooth muscle mass via direct application of thermal energy. Severe asthma is a widespread problem globally. There are 22.9 million Americans in the United States with asthma,[2] and severe persistent asthma constitutes up to 12%[3-5] yet disproportionately utilizes more direct and indirect health care dollars for asthma care.[6-8]

SEVERE ASTHMA

Severe persistent asthma consists of asthma symptoms throughout the day, nighttime awakenings often 7 times a week, need for short-acting β-agonists several times a day, and extreme limitations in daily activity as well as forced expiratory volume in 1 second (FEV_1) less than 60% predicted (without medications).[9] Risk factors for

All of the authors report no financial conflicts of interest in relation to the completion of this research.

Department of Medicine, The Ohio State University Wexner Medical Center, Columbus, OH, USA

* Corresponding author. 201 Davis Heart and Lung Institute, 473 West 12th Avenue, Columbus, OH 43210.

E-mail address: Karen.Wood@osumc.edu

Otolaryngol Clin N Am 47 (2014) 77–86
http://dx.doi.org/10.1016/j.otc.2013.09.007
oto.theclinics.com

Abbreviations	
AIR	Asthma Intervention Research
ASM	Airway smooth muscle
ATS	American Thoracic Society
BT	Bronchial thermoplasty
FEV$_1$	Forced expiratory volume in 1 second
LABA	Long-acting β-agonist

severe asthma include being female (postpuberty), obesity, black race, significant secondhand smoke exposure, and comorbidities of gastroesophageal reflux, sinus infections, and pneumonia.[10] Although control is the ultimate goal in the management of asthma, complete control in many with severe persistent asthma is often elusive,[11] leading to several terms to describe this patient group, including *severe asthma*, *steroid-dependent or resistant asthma*, *difficult or poorly controlled asthma*, and *brittle or irreversible asthma*.[12] In 2000, the "Proceedings of the ATS Workshop on Refractory Asthma" agreed on the term, *refractory asthma*, to describe those asthma cases requiring a high amount of medications to maintain control or those cases of persistent symptoms, airflow obstruction, and frequent exacerbations despite high medication use.[12] Diagnosis requires all other diseases with similar presenting symptoms to have been ruled out, comorbid conditions adequately managed, and medication technique and adherence issues addressed.[12]

The lack of therapeutic effectiveness or response to traditional medications in this patient group raises the question of differing airway pathophysiology compared with mild or moderate asthmatics[12] and has led to a discussion of asthma being a heterogeneous disease with varying manifestations or responses to treatment.[13] Several distinct phenotypes are evolving when comparing clinical and physiologic features, prominence of biomarkers, age of disease onset, and response to therapy; however, additional research is needed for full characterization.[10,14,15] The movement from symptom-based therapy decisions to medications or interventions targeting the underlying physiologic features of the disease will pave the way to personalized treatment plans, with the ultimate goal of improved control for refractory asthmatics.

PATHOPHYSIOLOGY

One important target of current asthma therapy is ASM because it is critically involved in asthma pathogenesis. Acutely, ASM cell contraction causes bronchoconstriction. Chronically, hypertrophy and hyperplasia of ASM are responsible for airway remodeling.[9] Additionally, through interactions with other cells, such as mast cells, and by generating and releasing inflammatory mediators, ASM cells are responsible for some of the airway inflammation seen with asthma.[16] Medications, such as short-acting bronchodilators, long-acting bronchodilators, leukotriene inhibitors, and theophylline, play an important role in asthma management by relaxing the ASM. BT is used as a new approach to treatment by structurally modifying the airway and destroying smooth muscle. If ASM is to be destroyed, it is important to believe that ASM does not have a physiologic role. Investigators have debated if ASM has a beneficial or physiologic role or whether it is similar to a vestigial organ and serves no useful purpose.[17] This debate has not been settled; many researchers and clinicians have proposed possible roles for ASM.[18] Refractory asthmatics present a crucial opportunity to better understand the underlying pathophysiology of asthma and the importance of targeting specific pathways for treatment. The complexity of the inflammatory cascade and chemoreceptors associated with asthma reduces the possibility of a single treatment approach for a cure. Although BT has been associated with reduced frequency of asthma exacerbations, some unknown factors persist because airway inflammation remains intact and medications remain necessary for management.

RESULTS AND EFFICACY
Preclinical Studies

In 2004, investigators published a study using radiofrequency ablation (BT) at 3 different temperatures in 11 dogs with some of the dogs followed as long as 3 years. The investigators found a significant reduction in airway hyperresponsiveness among the BT-treated (at 65°C or 75°C) versus untreated airways of the canines using local methacholine provocation directed to the treated airways.[19] Histologic evaluation of the canine airways (up to 3 years after treatment) showed persistent ASM reduction and no evidence of smooth muscle regeneration. This study also established a correlation between the extent of reduction in ASM and improvement in airway hyperresponsiveness. These results were subsequently validated in 3 additional canine studies.[20–22]

Human Studies

Lung cancer, no asthma
The first human feasibility study was conducted by Miller and colleagues.[23] Nine subjects without asthma but with known lung cancer scheduled to undergo surgical resection participated in this study; however, only 8 underwent BT. BT was targeted to visually accessible airway segments, which were planned for surgical resection. All subjects had an office follow-up visit in-between the BT treatment and surgery. All patients tolerated the procedure well and there were no procedure-related complications (including respiratory tract infections, need for additional medications, supplemental oxygen, and unscheduled health care visits). Histologic evaluation of both the treated and untreated tissue was performed. An approximately 50% reduction in ASM was noted in airways of those treated to 65°C versus a 5% reduction among persons treated to 55°C. The investigators concluded that BT is well tolerated among humans and yielded significant reduction in ASM mass.

Mild to moderate asthma
Subsequent studies were conducted evaluating BT in asthmatic patients (**Table 1**). The first was a nonrandomized prospective study of 16 patients with stable mild to moderate asthma[24]; 13 of the 16 subjects completed all 3 sessions and were followed for 2 years post-BT. There was a significant improvement in airway hyperresponsiveness but no improvement in FEV_1 after 2 years. BT was well tolerated among asthmatics; however, in comparison to the feasibility study, there were side effects. The most common adverse events were mild and consisted of

- Cough (94% of subjects)
- Chest discomfort (56%)
- Dyspnea (69%)
- Wheezing (50%)
- Bronchospasm (63%)
- Mucus production (50%)
- Fever (44%)

Table 1
Summary of bronchial thermoplasty clinical trials

Study	Study Design	Asthma Severity	Follow-up (y)	Improved Outcomes	Outcomes Without Change
Cox et al,[24]	Prospective nonrandomized	Mild to moderate, stable asthma	2	AHR Symptom-free days Morning PEF Evening PEF	FEV_1 Rescue medicine usage
Cox et al,[25]	Prospective randomized	Moderate to severe persistent asthma	1	Morning PEF Symptom-free days Quality-of-life scores Rescue medicine usage	AHR FEV_1
Pavord et al,[26]	Prospective randomized	Refractory asthma	1	Quality-of-life scores Rescue medicine usage Prebronchodilator FEV_1	AHR Symptom-free days Morning PEF Evening PEF Postbronchodilator FEV_1
Castro et al,[27]	Randomized, double-blind, sham-controlled	Severe persistent asthma	1	Severe asthma exacerbations ED visits Missed work/school days	Pre- or postbronchodilator FEV_1 Rescue medicine usage Symptom-free days Morning PEF

Abbreviations: AHR, airway hyperresponsiveness; ED, emergency department; PEF, peak expiratory flow.
Data from Refs.[24-27]

There were no postprocedure hospitalizations or severe adverse events related to BT.

The Asthma Intervention Research (AIR) Trial was the first randomized multicenter study evaluating BT[25]; 112 subjects with moderate to severe persistent asthma were enrolled and randomized to either inhaled corticosteroid with a long-acting β-agonist (LABA) or BT plus combination inhaled corticosteroid and LABA. Subjects were followed for 2 years. The study showed an improvement in asthma symptoms; however, no difference in airway hyperresponsiveness was observed. Adverse events were common immediately post-treatment in the BT cohort, with 4 subjects requiring hospitalization for asthma exacerbations. Again a majority of adverse events were mild and mainly consisted of cough, dyspnea, wheezing, and chest tightness. The major limitation of this study was its nonblinded study design and lack of sham control leading to a potential placebo effect.

Although the safety and efficacy of BT among mild, moderate, and severe persistent asthma had been evaluated, the question remained as to whether patients with refractory asthma could benefit from this novel asthma therapy. Pavord and colleagues[26] performed a randomized trial aimed at evaluating the efficacy of BT among symptomatic severe asthmatics; 34 subjects with refractory asthma were enrolled in this year-long, multinational study comparing BT with a control, medical management arm. Subjects in this study were on higher doses of inhaled corticosteroids and oral prednisone in comparison with previously published studies. At completion of the study, subjects in the BT arm had a significant reduction in use of short-acting β-agonist, improvement in prebronchodilator FEV_1, but not postbronchodilator FEV_1, and improved Asthma Control Questionnaire scores compared with subjects in the medical therapy arm. During the treatment period, 7 hospitalizations for respiratory symptoms occurred in 4 of the 15 BT patients compared with none in the control arm. Two hospitalizations were secondary to segmental collapse of the recently treated lobe whereas 5 were for asthma exacerbations. Aside from the treatment portion of the study, hospitalization rates were similar for the two groups.

Although each of these studies highlights efficacy, safety, and complications associated with BT among small and specific asthma populations, they had significant limitations. In 2010, the Asthma Intervention Research 2 Trial (AIR2) trial, a randomized, double-blinded, sham-controlled study, was published.[27] In order to achieve the double-blind design, subjects were evaluated by a blinded assessment team and treatments were conducted by an unblinded bronchoscopy team. The sham bronchoscopy used a sham radiofrequency controller, which was indistinguishable with the exception of no deliverable energy; 288 subjects with severe asthma were enrolled. The Asthma Quality of Life Questionnaire scores were significantly improvement from baseline in the BT group compared with the sham group. More remarkably, the study showed a significant reduction in severe exacerbations, emergency department visits, and missed work/school days post-BT. Adverse events were mostly mild to moderate in severity and consisted mainly of symptoms of airway inflammation. Again, the BT group had a higher postprocedure hospitalization rate (8.4%–2% of the sham group), and severe adverse events included 1 episode of hemoptysis requiring bronchial artery embolization.

Since the definitive study for BT by Castro and colleagues,[27] its use for the treatment of adults greater than or equal to 18 years with severe persistent asthma that is uncontrolled despite inhaled corticosteroids and LABA has been approved by the FDA. Despite FDA approval, its efficacy and safety continue to be studied. There are few data on the long-term benefits. Further research is needed to determine the long-term safety and efficacy of BT on asthma as well as specific patient selection recommendations to determine which asthma phenotypes respond the best to BT.

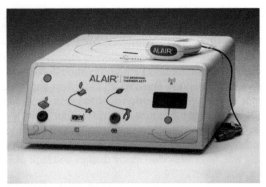

Fig. 1. The Alair Bronchial Thermoplasty System control unit with the catheter on top. (*Courtesy of* Boston Scientific Corporation, Natick, MA.)

TECHNIQUE

BT administers controlled radiofrequency waves to the airways using the Alair System (Boston Scientific, Natick, Massachusetts) (Video 1, **Fig. 1**), which consists of a radiofrequency generator and a disposable bronchial catheter with an expandable basket consisting of 4 electrodes. BT is typically performed via 3 bronchoscopy sessions spaced 3 weeks apart. Accessible distal airways of all lobes except the right middle lobe are treated (**Fig. 2**). Each lower lobe's airways are treated separately during 1 of the first 2 sessions. Both upper lobes are treated during the third and final session.[28]

Systemic steroids, usually prednisone (50 mg), are typically administered for 5 days starting 2 to 3 days prior to BT to minimize postprocedure inflammation. Preprocedure assessment typically includes establishment of baseline spirometry, screening to ensure no evidence of an acute asthma exacerbation or upper respiratory tract

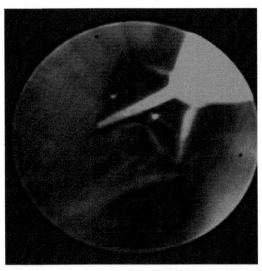

Fig. 2. The electrode basket is expanded in the airways, making contact with the wall for application of thermal energy.

infection, and administration of a short-acting bronchodilator just prior to the bronchoscopy. Once the preprocedure assessment has been completed and informed consent obtained, the patient is prepped for bronchoscopy.

A grounding pad is applied to the patient's torso and connected to the radiofrequency generator. Sedation for BT is accomplished with a combination of local anesthesia and either deep or moderate sedation. A standard adult bronchoscope is then advanced through the vocal cords and a detailed airway examination with particular attention to previously treated airways is completed. The procedure is aborted if signs of active infection or evidence of inadequate airway healing are seen. The bronchoscope is then advanced to the most distal airways of the targeted lobe(s) while maintaining view of the airway wall. Next the electrode basket is advanced through the working channel of the bronchoscope and expanded until it contacts the airway walls (see **Fig. 2**). After sufficient airway contact with the basket is ensured, the operator delivers 10 seconds[29] of thermal energy yielding a target tissue temperature of 65°C.[19,23] The electrode basket is then collapsed and retracted 5 mm to the site of the next treatment. This process is repeated in a distal to proximal fashion ensuring contiguous but nonoverlapping applications.[30] The on-line video clip (supplementary online data) demonstrates application of energy in a live procedure.

Each BT session lasts approximately 40 to 60 minutes.[29] A preprocedure treatment plan is crucial to ensure no airway segments undergo duplicate or missed treatments. Additionally, close monitoring of oxygenation during the procedure with supplemental oxygen less than fraction of inspired oxygen (Fio_2) less than 40% is needed to prevent airway fire. On completion of the session, the bronchoscope is removed and the patient closely monitored in recovery. Once the patient has recovered from sedation and the FEV_1 is 80% or greater of the preprocedure FEV_1, the patient may be discharged to home with close follow-up. Detailed instructions on when to contact the physician and schedule follow-up should be included in the postprocedure plan.

PRACTICAL APPLICATIONS
Patient Selection

The only approved indication for BT based on studies to date is severe asthma not adequately controlled with maximal medical therapy in patients over the age of 18. There are, however, several contraindications listed by the FDA. These include

- Presence of an implanted electronic device, such as a pacemaker or defibrillator
- Sensitivities to any of the medications necessary for bronchoscopy
- Patients previously treated with BT should not be treated again in the same area.

BT should also be deferred when any of these conditions is present:

- Active respiratory infection
- Asthma exacerbation within 2 weeks
- Coagulopathy
- Patient unable to stop taking anticoagulant medications

Because the AIR2 study was the definitive study, the inclusion and exclusion criteria used for this study should be kept in mind. Subjects were included between the ages of 18 and 65 years old diagnosed with asthma and requiring moderate to high doses of inhaled corticosteroids and a LABA. Subjects could be on other asthma maintenance medications, including oral corticosteroids, provided the dose was less than 10 mg/d. Stability on the medications was required for a minimum of 4 weeks prior to the procedure and the subjects had prebronchodilator FEV_1 60% or greater predicted as well as documentation of airway hyperresponsiveness through methacholine challenge. Additionally, the subjects were nonsmoking for at least 1 year with no more than a 10 pack/y smoking history and at least 2 days of asthma symptoms during the preceding 4 weeks.[27] Key exclusion criteria were life-threatening asthma (intubated for asthma during their lifetime, hospitalized in intensive care within the previous 24 months, more than 3 asthma exacerbations requiring hospitalizations, 3 or more lower respiratory infections, or 4 steroid bursts in the previous 12 months); chronic sinus disease; other respiratory disease, such as emphysema; and use of immunosuppressants, β-adrenergic blocking agents, anticoagulants, or implanted electrical devices.[27]

Follow-Up

Patients should be followed closely after the procedure to monitor for adverse events associated with BT (**Table 2**). Although there is no standard established follow-up, one schedule entails contacting the patients by phone several times after the procedure (1, 2, and 7 days after the procedure, for example) followed by an office visit 2 weeks after each BT session. Because a majority of adverse events occur closely after BT, patients may resume their normal follow-up schedule for severe asthma after the 2-week visit.

Potential Safety Concerns

BT remains controversial among providers for refractory asthmatics in part because of few data on long-term safety and effectiveness and less specificity in knowing which severe asthma phenotypes are more likely to benefit.[31] Also concerning is the applicability of BT to this patient group because a result of the strict inclusion and exclusion criteria used in the initial trials would have excluded many refractory asthmatics.[27] In the first feasibility study in human subjects, treated airways showed approximately 50% reduction in the smooth muscle mass (2 weeks post-treatment); however, this has not correlated with improvements in FEV_1 in subjects evaluated in the effectiveness and safety studies, suggesting additional inquiry is needed to fully understand the physiologic effect in the post-BT airway.[23,25,31–33] Case reports and larger formal studies mandated by the FDA are forthcoming and may help clarify these issues.[1] In the interim, safety studies have been reassuring up to 5 years postprocedure with stable lung function, consistently higher quality-of-life scores, and reduced exacerbations in treated subjects, offering a novel treatment option to those who are significantly limited by their disease.[25,27,33,34]

Table 2 Potential adverse events associated with bronchial thermoplasty and in the postprocedure period	
Wheezing	Cough
Chest discomfort	Dyspnea
Sputum production	Nasal/chest congestion
Bronchospasm	Night awakenings
Respiratory tract infections	Atelectasis
Throat irritation/pain	Hypoxia
Fever	Hemoptysis

SUMMARY

BT is a novel therapy for severe asthma. It involves 3 separate bronchoscopic procedures spaced 3 weeks apart. During the procedure, radiofrequency waves are applied to the airways. The procedure results in decreased asthma symptoms and exacerbations and an increased quality of life. Pathologically, the application of thermal energy results in a reduction of ASM, which is believed the basis for symptomatic improvement. Complications can develop from the procedure, however, and patients need to be chosen carefully and followed closely afterward.

SUPPLEMENTARY DATA

Supplementary video related to this article is found at http://dx.doi.org/10.1016/j.otc. 2013.09.007. (*Video;* Courtesy of Boston Scientific Corporation, Natick, MA).

REFERENCES

1. Alair Bronchial Thermoplasty System -P080032. 2010 May 19, 2010 [cited 2013 June 21]; Available from: http://www.accessdata.fda.gov/cdrh_docs/pdf8/ P080032b.pdf.
2. American Lung Association Lung Disease Data: 2008. 2008 [cited 2013 June 21]; Available from: http://www.lung.org/assets/documents/publications/lung-disease-data/LDD_2008.pdf.
3. Birnbaum HG, Ivanova JI, Yu AP, et al. Asthma severity categorization using a claims-based algorithm or pulmonary function testing. J Asthma 2009;46: 67–72.
4. Michelson PH, Williams LW, Benjamin DK, et al. Obesity, inflammation, and asthma severity in childhood: data from the National Health and Nutrition Examination Survey 2001-2004. Ann Allergy Asthma Immunol 2009;103:381–5.
5. Clark NM, Dodge JA, Shah S, et al. A current picture of asthma diagnosis, severity, and control in a low-income minority preteen population. J Asthma 2010;47:150–5.
6. Cisternas MG, Blanc PD, Yen IH, et al. A comprehensive study of the direct and indirect costs of adult asthma. J Allergy Clin Immunol 2003;111:1212–8.
7. Ivanova JI, Bergman R, Birnbaum HG, et al. Effect of asthma exacerbations on health care costs among asthmatic patients with moderate and severe persistent asthma. J Allergy Clin Immunol 2012;129:1229–35.
8. Szefler SJ, Zeiger RS, Haselkorn T, et al. Economic burden of impairment in children with severe or difficult-to-treat asthma. Ann Allergy Asthma Immunol 2011; 107:110–9.e111.
9. National Asthma Education and Prevention Program. Expert Panel Report 3 (EPR-3): Guidelines for the Diagnosis and Management of Asthma-Summary Report 2007. J Allergy Clin Immunol 2007;120:S94–138.
10. Jarjour NN, Erzurum SC, Bleecker ER, et al. Severe asthma: lessons learned from the National Heart, Lung, and Blood Institute Severe Asthma Research Program. Am J Respir Crit Care Med 2012;185:356–62.
11. Chipps BE, Zeiger RS, Borish L, et al. Key findings and clinical implications from The Epidemiology and Natural History of Asthma: Outcomes and Treatment Regimens (TENOR) study. J Allergy Clin Immunol 2012;130:332–42.e310.
12. Proceedings of the ATS workshop on refractory asthma: current understanding, recommendations, and unanswered questions. American Thoracic Society. Am J Respir Crit Care Med 2000;162:2341–51.

13. Bousquet J, Mantzouranis E, Cruz AA, et al. Uniform definition of asthma severity, control, and exacerbations: document presented for the World Health Organization Consultation on Severe Asthma. J Allergy Clin Immunol 2010;126:926–38.

14. Wenzel SE. Asthma phenotypes: the evolution from clinical to molecular approaches. Nat Med 2012;18:716–25.

15. Carolan BJ, Sutherland ER. Clinical phenotypes of chronic obstructive pulmonary disease and asthma: recent advances. J Allergy Clin Immunol 2013;131:627–34 [quiz: 635].

16. Black JL, Panettieri RA Jr, Banerjee A, et al. Airway smooth muscle in asthma: just a target for bronchodilation? Clin Chest Med 2012;33:543–58.

17. Mitzner W. Airway smooth muscle: the appendix of the lung. Am J Respir Crit Care Med 2004;169:787–90.

18. Panettieri RA Jr, Kotlikoff MI, Gerthoffer WT, et al. Airway smooth muscle in bronchial tone, inflammation, and remodeling: basic knowledge to clinical relevance. Am J Respir Crit Care Med 2008;177:248–52.

19. Danek CJ, Lombard CM, Dungworth DL, et al. Reduction in airway hyperresponsiveness to methacholine by the application of RF energy in dogs. J Appl Physiol 2004;97:1946–53.

20. Brown R, Wizeman W, Danek C, et al. Effect of bronchial thermoplasty on airway closure. Clin Med Circ Respirat Pulm Med 2007;1:1–6.

21. Brown RH, Wizeman W, Danek C, et al. Effect of bronchial thermoplasty on airway distensibility. Eur Respir J 2005;26:277–82.

22. Brown RH, Wizeman W, Danek C, et al. In vivo evaluation of the effectiveness of bronchial thermoplasty with computed tomography. J Appl Physiol 2005;98:1603–6.

23. Miller JD, Cox G, Vincic L, et al. A prospective feasibility study of bronchial thermoplasty in the human airway. Chest 2005;127:1999–2006.

24. Cox G, Miller JD, McWilliams A, et al. Bronchial thermoplasty for asthma. Am J Respir Crit Care Med 2006;173:965–9.

25. Cox G, Thomson NC, Rubin AS, et al. Asthma control during the year after bronchial thermoplasty. N Engl J Med 2007;356:1327–37.

26. Pavord ID, Cox G, Thomson NC, et al. Safety and efficacy of bronchial thermoplasty in symptomatic, severe asthma. Am J Respir Crit Care Med 2007;176:1185–91.

27. Castro M, Rubin AS, Laviolette M, et al. Effectiveness and safety of bronchial thermoplasty in the treatment of severe asthma: a multicenter, randomized, double-blind, sham-controlled clinical trial. Am J Respir Crit Care Med 2010;181:116–24.

28. Cox PG, Miller J, Mitzner W, et al. Radiofrequency ablation of airway smooth muscle for sustained treatment of asthma: preliminary investigations. Eur Respir J 2004;24:659–63.

29. Cox G. Bronchial thermoplasty. Clin Chest Med 2010;31:135–40. Table of Contents.

30. Mayse ML, Rubin A, Lampron N, et al. Clinical pearls for bronchial thermoplasty. Journal of Bronchology & Interventional Pulmonology 2007;14:115–23.

31. Wahidi MM, Kraft M. Bronchial thermoplasty for severe asthma. Am J Respir Crit Care Med 2012;185:709–14.

32. Cayetano KS, Chan AL, Albertson TE, et al. Bronchial thermoplasty: a new treatment paradigm for severe persistent asthma. Clin Rev Allergy Immunol 2012;43:184–93.

33. Thomson NC, Rubin AS, Niven RM, et al. Long-term (5 year) safety of bronchial thermoplasty: Asthma Intervention Research (AIR) trial. BMC Pulm Med 2011;11:8.

34. Doeing DC, Mahajan AK, White SR, et al. Safety and feasibility of bronchial thermoplasty in asthma patients with very severe fixed airflow obstruction: a case series. J Asthma 2013;50:215–8.

The Role of Fractional Exhaled Nitric Oxide in Asthma Management

Karen H. Calhoun, MD

KEYWORDS

- Fractional exhaled nitric oxide • Allergic inflammation • Asthma management
- Lung function

KEY POINTS

- Clinical management of asthma is challenging, and measuring exhaled nitric oxide can provide another type of data to assist in meeting this challenge.
- Fractional exhaled nitric oxide (FeNO) is relatively easy to perform, and the equipment is not forbiddingly expensive.
- FeNO provides a complement to traditional measures of asthma control and can help guide diagnostic and treatment choices.

FENO: WHY SHOULD I CARE?

Short answer: *It may help manage your asthmatic patients.*

The challenges of asthma care include[1]: Does this patient have asthma (**Figs. 1** and **2**)?[2] How severe is the asthma?[3] What medications will help this patient most?[4] Is this patient improving or getting worse?[5] Is this patient compliant with his/her medications?[6] Is this patient at current risk for an asthma exacerbation?

Traditional methods for answering these questions include symptom questionnaires, peak flow measurements, spirometry, eosinophil count in induced sputum, bronchoalveolar lavage (BAL) fluid or biopsy,[1] and spirometric methacholine challenge. The problems with these methods are subjectivity (questionnaire), dependence on patient voluntary performance (peak flow, spirometry, and methacholine challenge), invasiveness (induced sputum, BAL, and biopsy), and time and complexity of performing them (all except questionnaires and peak flow). There is, therefore, a continual search for quick and easy objective measurements to help with asthma diagnosis and management.

Department of Otolaryngology - Head & Neck Surgery, Wexner Medical Center, The Ohio State University College of Medicine, Columbus, OH, USA
E-mail address: karen.calhoun@osumc.edu

Otolaryngol Clin N Am 47 (2014) 87–96
http://dx.doi.org/10.1016/j.otc.2013.09.001
0030-6665/14/$ – see front matter © 2014 Elsevier Inc. All rights reserved.

Abbreviations	
AR	Allergic rhinitis
BAL	Bronchoalveolar lavage
BHR	Bronchial hyperreactivity
COPD	Chronic obstructive pulmonary disease
EIB	Exercise-induced bronchospasm
FeNO	Fractional exhaled nitric oxide
FEV_1	Forced expiratory volume in the first second of expiration
ICS	Inhaled corticosteroid
NAR	Nonallergic rhinitis
NO	Nitric oxide
NOS	Nitric oxide synthase
PEF	Peak expiratory flow
SAR	Seasonal allergic rhinitis

WHAT IS FENO?

Short answer: *FeNO is a marker for eosinophilic inflammation in the lungs.*

FeNO a marker for inflammation that can be measured in the exhaled breath. Human airways respond to inflammation by producing nitric oxide (NO) via nitric oxide synthase (NOS). NOS2A isoform is produced by cells in the bronchial wall, and this mechanism overproduces NO when there is eosinophilic inflammation.[2,3] It is being investigated as an objective measure to assist with asthma management.

The first machines for measuring exhaled NO depended on chemiluminescence analyzers and were fairly large and nonportable. Currently, most clinical offices in the

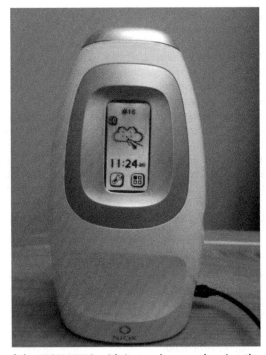

Fig. 1. Front view of the NIOX MINO with its touchscreen showing the cloud graphic.

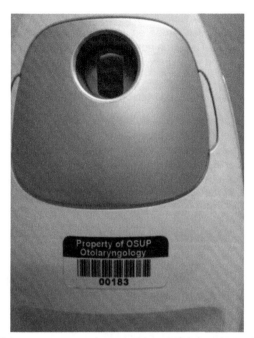

Fig. 2. Back view of the NIOX MINO. The opening toward the top is where the disposable mouthpiece is inserted. Because the patient blows from the back and the graphic is on the front, it is easiest the have the patient watch the touchscreen in a mirror. There is also an audio cue, with a steady sound for acceptable inhalation speed and a high-pitched beeping when the speed is too slow or too fast.

United States use the NIOX MINO (Aerocrine AB), which measures FeNO by an electrochemical analyzer. The handheld machine has a disposable mouthpiece that is changed between patients. Because concentration of NO depends on the speed of exhalation, the NIOX MINO is calibrated to a preferred flow rate of 50 mL/s.[4] It has a sensitivity and reproducibility of 1 ppb, with a range of 1 ppb to 500 ppb. Patients are instructed to exhale deeply, place their mouth on the mouthpiece, and inhale deeply through the mouthpiece. This inhalation through the built-in filter screens out NO in the inhaled breath. Immediately after inhalation, patients exhale at a slow, steady rate, holding near 50 mL/s for 10 seconds. There is a floating cloud on the machine that provides video game–like instant feedback to patients. Additionally, an on-computer module add-on is available that is even more engaging, featuring a hot-air balloon flying over water between two land masses.[4,5]

FeNO measurement is noninvasive, easy, and simple to perform. Most patients, including young children, are able to perform it correctly with a bit of coaching (much less extensive than that required for reliable spirometry). The exhalation needed for FeNO is gentle, like blowing on soup to cool it, rather than the prolonged forceful exhalation required for spirometry, so it is easier for the elderly and the ill. The equipment is inexpensive and easy to maintain.

Asthmatic patients not on inhaled corticosteroids (ICSs) often have elevated FeNO readings. The manufacturer of the NIOX MINO recommends that values under 25 (20 for children) be regarded as normal, those between 25 and 50 (20–40 for children) as intermediate, and values over 50 (40 for children) as abnormally high.

Some of the initial enthusiasm about the potential usefulness of FeNO in diagnosing and managing asthma has been tempered as reports accrue identifying other pathologies also affecting FeNO.[6] The remainder of this article summarizes current findings and thoughts about how and when FeNO can be useful in the management of asthma.

WHAT ELSE AFFECTS FENO MEASUREMENT?

Short answer: *FeNO is affected by multiple demographic and lifestyle issues.*

FeNO is affected by genetic phenotypes, age and gender, race, possibly height and weight, and definitely the presence of atopic disease or current upper respiratory tract infection. FeNO is higher in males than females and higher in adults than children. It is higher in Chinese schoolchildren and African American adults than in white populations of similar ages.[7–12]

Vigorous exercise prior to FeNO measurement can produce falsely low levels.[10]

Spirometry before FeNO may or may not have a similar effect.[10,13] Breath-holding increases FeNO.[4] Depression and prolonged stress can lower FeNO levels.[14] Acute exposure to moderate altitude significantly increased FeNO by approximately 20%.[15] Increased air pollution is associated with higher FeNO. Specifically, diesel exhaust increases FeNO in a laboratory setting, but ozone does not.[2,16] Allergy immunotherapy decreases FeNO.[17]

It is recommended that patients do not eat or drink for an hour before testing. Specifically, alcohol, like smoking, decreases FeNO, and nitrate-containing foods, such as bacon or lettuce, transiently increase FeNO.[4,10]

Sordillo and colleagues[8] studied children, finding that allergy to indoor antigens was associated with increased FeNO. Additionally, watching more than 10 hours of television during the weekdays of each week was associated with increased FeNO even after controlling for indoor allergen exposure, allergic sensitization, and body mass index. They concluded that sedentary behavior might be another independent factor capable of increasing FeNO.

WHAT OTHER DISEASES AFFECT FENO?

Short answer: *FeNO is affected by several other pulmonary pathologies as well as some nonpulmonary ones.*

FeNO is abnormally low in pulmonary hypertension, cystic fibrosis, HIV infection, and primary ciliary dyskinesia.[18] It is relatively low in stable bronchiectasis.[19] FeNO has been found significantly elevated in patients with acute eosinophilic pneumonia.[20]

Obstructive sleep apnea is associated with higher oral NO and FeNO levels. These tend to decrease after appropriate continuous positive airway pressure treatment.[21,22]

HOW GOOD IS FENO AS A SCREEN FOR ASTHMA?

Short answer: *There is contradictory evidence, with some studies showing excellent correlation, and others showing no correlation. Overall consensus seems that FeNO may be useful screening for asthma in patients with allergic rhinitis (AR) and/or respiratory symptoms.*

Investigations of rhinitis patients and population-based studies have demonstrated that many people have subclinical bronchial hyperreactivity (BHR).[20] BHR is associated with future development of AR and asthma.[23] If there were a way to identify not only patients with undiagnosed or undertreated frank asthma but also those with subclinical lower airway inflammation who are at risk of developing reactive airway disease or asthma, these patients could be targeted with more-aggressive treatment.

Lee and colleagues[20] investigated using FeNO to screen for asthma in Chinese schoolchildren. They measured FeNO in controls and in children with physician-diagnosed AR and/or asthma and/or atopic dermatitis. They showed that asthma and AR were independently associated with increases in FeNO, concluding that "other diseases besides asthma should be considered when applying FeNO as a screening tool for asthma..." It may be accurate to draw another conclusion from their data: that FeNO screening of patients with AR and no history of asthma can identify those who should have further work-up for asthma.

Ciprandi and colleagues[24] found that children with AR or asthma who had FeNO greater than 34 ppb were more likely to have reversibility after bronchodilator administration, especially if they were also sensitized to perennial allergens. This suggests that both FeNO and pattern of allergen exposure can help guide identification of children who would benefit from further pulmonary work-up.

Schleich and colleagues[25] examined how well FeNO or forced expiratory volume in the first second of expiration (FEV_1) less than 101% predicted a positive outcome to a methacholine challenge in steroid-naive patients with respiratory symptoms. Inhaled methacholine stimulates bronchoconstriction, with a decrease of 20% or more generally regarded as indicating asthma. They found that a FeNO greater than 34 ppb had a positive predictive value of 88%, specificity of 95%, sensitivity of 35%, and negative predictive value of 662% with respect to a positive methacholine challenge. Because methacholine challenge is a time-consuming complex test compared with FeNO, there may be a role for FeNO in screening for early asymptomatic BHR, permitting closer follow-up of those who are at higher risk for developing respiratory disease.[26]

Ciebiada and colleagues[26] also looked at patients with seasonal AR (SAR) and no asthma, comparing them with normal controls. All had FeNO, nasal congestion scores, and nasal peak inspiratory flow measured 6 weeks before pollen season, at the height of pollen season, and 6 weeks after pollen season. SAR patients had higher FeNO preseason, and FeNO increased in both groups in pollen season, but was a significant increase only in the SAR group. This confirms that exposure to allergens tends to increase FeNO.

Fukuhara and colleagues[27] screened patients presenting with cough, wheeze, or dyspnea. When traditional screening methods for asthma were compared with FeNO, a FeNO greater than 40 had 78.6% sensitivity and 89.5% specificity for identifying asthma. These investigators mention the necessity of excluding other pulmonary pathologies but concluded that FeNO screen for asthma was effective in such a population for screening in daily clinical practice.

Kakoaklioglu and colleagues[28] screened FeNO levels in 5 groups: controls without rhinitis and patients with non-AR (NAR) and AR, with or without asthma. FeNO was, as expected, lowest in controls and NAR without asthma. The FeNO levels in AR patients with or without asthma were, as expected, higher than in NAR patients without asthma or the controls. But the highest levels occurred in asthmatic patients with rhinitis, whether AR or NAR. These investigators concluded that whether a patient has rhinitis or not was a stronger influence on increasing FeNO that whether the rhinitis is allergic in nature or not.

ElHalawani and colleagues[29] studied patients without a history of asthma, atopy, or smoking referred for evaluation of possible exercise-induced bronchospasm (EIB), which used to be called exercise-induced asthma. Sometimes presumed EIB is treated empirically with a pre-exercise inhaled bronchodilator; when, however, the precise cause of exertional dyspnea is unclear, spirometry measurement before and after 6 to 8 minutes of treadmill or similar exercise is required. This group's focus was whether FeNO (faster, easier, and less expensive) could obviate some of this exercise testing. They measured FeNO before exercise and every 5 minutes for 30 minutes of exercise. They found that no patients with an initial FeNO of less than 12 ppb had EIB demonstrated by this spirometry. Specifically, in terms of effectiveness in excluding EIB, a FeNO less than 12 had a sensitivity of 1.0, a specificity of 0.31, a negative predictive value of 0.19, and a positive predictive value of 1.0. This finding suggests that patients presenting with exertional dyspnea and a FeNO less than 12 ppb can be spared exercise spirometry, with attention directed to other possible causes of this dyspnea.

Buchwald and colleagues[30] used a similar strategy in screening asthmatic children for EIB. Their group found that children with a FeNO less than 20 (or less than 12 if they were currently on ICSs) had only 1 chance in 10 of having concurrent EIB. They conclude, "Measurement of FeNO is a simple, and time- and resource-efficient tool that may be used to screen for EIB testing and therefore optimizes the resources for exercise testing in pediatric asthma monitoring."[30]

A study of Mexican children with persistent asthma showed that a FeNO over 20 was associated with poorer asthma control and lung function. Such screening could provide an opportunity for intensified environmental and pharmaceutical intervention to prevent future exacerbations.[31]

In a primary care setting, in a group of children with AR and with or without asthma, FeNO was associated with house dust mite sensitization but not with nasal or asthma symptoms or rhinitis-related quality of life.[32]

My take from these studies is that FeNO provides useful screening for patients with AR and that levels over approximately 40 ppb, probably over 35 ppb in children, should prompt a further look at the possibility of BHR or asthma.

CAN FENO ASSIST IN CHOOSING APPROPRIATE MEDICATIONS?

Short answer: *Yes, those with high FeNO generally respond well to ICSs.*

In general, high FeNO (greater than 45 ppb) is associated with anticipated improvement with ICS therapy, including improvement in spirometry and BHR. A FeNO less than 25 ppb has been shown to have an 85% predictive value for absence of airway eosinophilc inflammation in adults.[3,10]

Clinically, there is a modest overlap between chronic obstructive pulmonary disease (COPD) and asthma, with some COPD patients showing BHR and responsiveness to ICSs. FeNO could be useful in suggesting which COPD patients are more likely to improve with ICSs, therefore deserving of a trial of this therapy.[30]

IS FENO USEFUL FOR ASSESSING PATIENT COMPLIANCE AND CONTROL?

Short answer: *Maybe, although this may be true only in select subpopulations of asthmatic patients.*

In many studies, FeNO increases as asthma worsens.[10] Matsunaga and colleagues[33] studied 250 stable asthmatics. They defined poor asthma control as an asthma control test score less than 20, or an FEV_1 or peak expiratory flow (PEF) less than 80% of predicted. They found that a FeNO greater than 39.5 could identify poorly controlled patients with 67% sensitivity and 76% specificity.[33] Another study (Gelb and colleagues'[34]) found that asthma patients with a FeNO greater than 28 ppb and an $FEV_{1\%}$ less than 76% of predicted had an 85% chance of asthma exacerbation over the next 18 months. There were zero exacerbations in patients with a FeNO less than 28 ppb and an $FEV_{1\%}$ greater than 76%.

In Nittner-Marxzalska and colleagues' study,[35] FeNO does not seem useful for monitoring pregnant asthmatics. There is, however, evidence that using FeNO to adjust ICS dose in nonpregnant patients can decrease the total amount of steroids needed for good disease control.[36]

Shaw and colleagues[37] compared management of asthma using FeNO to using the British Thoracic Society guidelines, which are based on history and spirometry response to bronchodilator of PEF or FEV_1. Using FeNO did not reduce the total dose of ICSs nor did it decrease the number of exacerbations. The investigators believed, however, that using FeNO to guide asthma therapy was feasible, just not superior to the BTS.

CAN FOLLOWING FENO ANTICIPATE EXACERBATIONS AND HELP PREVENT THEM?

Short answer: *Maybe, but further work is needed to define this.*

A 2009 Cochrane review examined the published evidence for whether FeNO works better than symptoms or spirometry for tailoring asthma treatment. It conclude that the benefit from using FeNO for this purpose is "modest at best" and does not recommend it.[38] A 2012 review by the same group looked at whether using FeNO or eosinophil count in induced sputum to guide treatment adjustments was better than traditional methods (symptoms, peak flow, and spirometry). They concluded that sputum eosinophil count was effective but not recommended routinely because of its invasiveness and that FeNO was not effective for this purpose.[1]

A 2013 article, however, performed a meta-analysis of the two adult studies examined in the 2012 report above plus one additional one. The investigators compared the use of symptoms alone versus symptoms and FeNO to guide treatment and concluded, "the rate of exacerbations was significantly reduced in favor of FeNO-based asthma management."[39]

van der Valk and colleagues[40] retrospectively examined 30 weeks of daily FeNO records of 77 children with asthma. During these 30 weeks there were 25 moderate and 12 severe exacerbations (severe = needing oral steroids, emergency department visit, or hospitalization). Moderate exacerbations were defined by the daily symptom score: 3 points above personal average score at least twice during a 2-week period or 5 points above at least once. For the moderate exacerbations, FeNO started to climb approximately 10 days beforehand. For the severe reactions, however, although FeNO increased, there was no such clear pattern. Because the severe reactions are the most medically significant, this was disappointing.

Spencer and colleagues[41] found that in asthmatic children not on ICSs, higher FeNO predicted greater need for a rescue inhaler both at the time of the study and 3 months hence. There was no such pattern for the children currently on ICSs.

BOTTOM LINE

The 2009 consensus statement from National Jewish Health concluded that appropriate uses for FeNO included showing the presence or absence of eosinophilic airway disease, estimating the chance of steroid responsiveness, assessing response to steroid treatment, and monitoring individual ICS compliance and estimating allergen exposure. They caution, however, that FeNO should not be used alone to diagnose asthma.[3]

FeNO may be most useful in patients with symptoms suggesting asthma. In these, a high FeNO suggests an allergic asthma etiology, and a low FeNO suggests a different pulmonary process was responsible for the symptoms.[10]

Because there is wide variability of FeNO among patient populations but stable findings in one person over time, one of the best uses of FeNO may be following an individual patient.[2]

The greatest value of FeNO in my practice is screening AR patients. A high FeNO reading, in patients with or without known asthma, is followed with prealbuterol and postalbuterol spirometry to assess lung function and BHR. Allergy skin testing is postponed if there is significant obstructive pulmonary disease, especially if combined with BHR. This provides an important safety function because one of the two main risk factors for a serious reaction to allergy skin testing is poorly controlled asthma. A high FeNO is expected to fall after initiation of ICS therapy, so failure to decrease as expected gives a signal to consider whether additional testing and consideration of alternate diagnoses are indicated. In addition, I retest patients with moderate or severe exacerbations of their AR symptoms as a gauge to help decide on further pharmacotherapy. Having FeNO available has provided sufficient information to make a mark.

There are now approximately 3000 articles in the world medical literature about FeNO and pulmonary processes. As the deluge of articles reporting fresh research continues, the answer to many of these questions will become clearer.

REFERENCES

1. Petsky HL, Caes CJ, Lasserson RJ, et al. A systematic review and meta-analysis: tailoring asthma treatment on eosinophilic markers (exhaled nitric oxide or sputum eosinophils). Thorax 2012;67:199–208.
2. La Grutta S, Ferrante G, Malizia V, et al. Environmental effects on fractional exhaled nitric oxide in allergic children. J Allergy (Cairo) 2012;2012:916926. http://dx.doi.org/10.1155/2012/916926, 6 pages.
3. Consensus statement of the use of fractional exhaled nitric oxide (FENO) in the clinical management of asthma. National Jewish Health; 2009.
4. American Thoracic Society, European Respiratory Society. American Thoracic Society Recommendations for standardized procedures for the online and offline measurement of exhaled lower respiratory nitric oxide and nasal nitric oxide. Am J Respir Crit Care Med 2005;171:912–30.
5. Xu F, Zou Z, Yan S, et al. Fractional exhaled nitric oxide in relation to asthma, allergic rhinitis and atopic dermatitis in Chinese children. J Asthma 2011;48: 1001–6.
6. Gevorgyan A, Fokkens WJ. Fractional exhaled nitric oxide (FeNO) measurement in asthma and rhinitis. Prim Care Respir J 2013;22(1):10–1.
7. Dweik RA, Boggs PB, Erzurum SC, et al. An official ATS clinical practice guideline: interpretation of exhaled nitric oxide levels (FeNO) for clinical applications. Am J Respir Crit Care Med 2011;184:602–15.
8. Sordillo JE, Webb T, Kwan D, et al. Allergen exposure modifies the relation of sensitization to fraction of exhaled nitric oxide levels in children at risk for allergy and asthma. J Allergy Clin Immunol 2011;127:1165–72.
9. Levesque MC, Hauswirth DW, Mervin-Blake S, et al. Deerminants of exhaled nitric oxide levels in healthy nonsmoking african american adults. J Allergy Clin Immunol 2008;121:396–402.
10. Barnes PJ, Dweik RA, Gelb AF, et al. Exhaled nitric oxide in pulmonary diseases: a comprehensive review. Chest 2010;138:682–92.
11. Hauswirth DW, Sundy JS, Mervin-Blake S, et al. Normative values for exhaled breath condensate pH and its relationship to exhaled nitric oxide in healthy African Americans. J Allergy Clin Immunol 2008;122:101–6.

12. Ishizuka T, Matsuzaki S, Aoki H, et al. Prevalence of asthma symptoms based on the European Community Respiratory Health Survey questionnsaire and FeNO in university students: gender difference in symptoms and FeNO. Allergy Asthma Clin Immunol 2011;7:15–23.
13. Prieto L, Ruiz-Jimenex L, Marin J. The effect of spirometry on bronchial and alveolar nitric oxide in subjects with asthma. J Asthma 2013;50(6):623–8.
14. Trueba AF, Smith NB, Auchus RJ, et al. Academic exam stress and depressive mood are associated with reductions in exhaled nitric oxide in healthy individuals. Biol Psychol 2013;93:206–12.
15. Caspersen C, Stang J, Thorsen E, et al. Exhaled nitric oxide concentration upon acute exposure to moderate altitude. Scand J Med Sci Sports 2013;23:102–7.
16. Barath S, Mills NL, Adelroth E, et al. Diesel exhaust but not ozine increases fraction of exhaled nitric oxide ina randomized controlled experimental exposure stufy of healthy huma subjects. Environ Health 2013;12:36.
17. Swiebocka EM, Siergiejko P, Rapeijko P, et al. Allergenic immunotherapy and seasonal changes in nitric oxide concentration in exhaled air in seasonal rhinitis patients. J Aerosol Med Pulm Drug Deliv 2012;25:1–5.
18. Khan S. The pitfalls of FeNO testing. Allergol Int 2013;62:143.
19. Cho YF, Lim HJ, Park JS, et al. Measurement of fractional exhaled nitric oxide in stable bronchiectasis. Tuberc Respir Dis (Seoul) 2013;74:7–14.
20. Lee JE, Rhee CK, Lim JH, et al. Fraction of exhaled nitric oxide in patients with acute eosinophilic pneumonia. Chest 2012;141(5):1267–72.
21. Culla B, Guida G, Brussino L, et al. Increased oral nitric oxide in OSA. Respir Med 2010;104:316–20.
22. Chua AP, Aboussouan LS, Minai OA, et al. Long term continuous positive airway pressure therapy normalizeds high exhaled nitric oxide levels in obstructive sleep apnea. J Clin Sleep Med 2013;9:529–35.
23. Marcon A, Cerveri I, Wjst M, et al. Can an airway challenge test predict respiratory diseases? A population-based international study. J Allergy Clin Immunol 2013; 2013. http://dx.doi.org/10.1016/j.jaci.2013.03.040. pii:S0091–6749(13)00529-0.
24. Ciprandi G, Tosca MA, Capasso M. High exhaled nitric oxide levels may predict bronchial reversibility in allergi children with asthma or rhinitis. J Asthma 2013;50:33–8.
25. Schleich FN, Asandei R, Manise M, et al. Is FENO50 useful diagnostic tool in suspected asthma? Int J Clin Pract 2012;66:158–65.
26. Ciebiada M, Cichocki P, Kasztalska K, et al. Orally exhaled nitric oxide in patients with seasonal allergic rhinitis during natural pollen season. Am J Rhinol Allergy 2012;26:e32–6.
27. Fukuhara A, Saito J, Sato S, et al. Validation study of asthma screening criteria based on subjective symptoms and fractional exhaled nitric oxide. Ann Allergy Asthma Immunol 2011;107:480–6.
28. Kakoaklioglu AF, Kalkan IK. Comparison of orally exhaled nitric oxide in allergic versus nonallergic rhinitis. Am J Rhinol Allergy 2012;26:e50–4. http://dx.doi.org/10.2500/ajra.2012.26.371.
29. ElHalawani SM, Ly NT, Mahon RT, et al. Exhaled nitric oxide as a predictor of exercise-induced bronchospasm. Chest 2003;124:639–43.
30. Buchwald F, Nermansen MN, Nielsen KG, et al. Exhaled nitric oxide predicts exercise-induced bronchospasm in asthmatic school children. Chest 2005;128:1964–7.
31. Soto-Ramos M, Castro-Rodriquez JA, Hinojos-Gallardo LC, et al. Fractional exhaled nitric oxide has good correlation with asthma control and lung function in Latino children with asthma. J Asthma 2013;50(6):590–4.

32. de Bot CM, Moed H, Bindels PJ, et al. Exhaled nitric oxide measures allergy in symptoms in children with allergic rhinitis in primary care: a prospective cross-sectional and longitudinal cohort study. Prim Care Respir J 2013;22:44–50.
33. Matsunaga K, Yanagisawa S, Hirano T, et al. Associated demographics of persistent exhaled nitric oxide elevation in treated asthmatics. Clin Exp Allergy 2011;42: 775–85.
34. Gelb AF, Flynn Taylor C, Shinar CM, et al. Role of spirometry and exhaled nitric oxide to predict exacerbations in treated asthmatics. Chest 2006;129:1492–9.
35. Nittner-Marxzalska M, Liebhart J, Pawlowicz R, et al. Fractioned exhaled nitric oxide (FENO) is not a sufficiently reliable test for monitoring asthma in pregnancy. Nitric Oxide 2013. http://dx.doi.org/10.1016/j.niox.2013.06.001. pii:S1089–8603(13)00155-9.
36. Smith AD, Cowan JO, Brassett KP, et al. Use of exhaled nitric oxide measurements to guide treatment in chronic asthma. N Engl J Med 2005;352:2163–73.
37. Shaw DE, Berry MA, Thomas M, et al. The use of exhaled nitric oxide to guide asthma management. A randomized controlled trial. Am J Respir Crit Care Med 2007;176:231–7.
38. Petsky HL, Cates CJ, Li A, et al. (Cochrane Airways Group) Tailored interventions based on exhaled nitric oxide versus clinical symptoms for asthma in children and adults [review]. Cochrane Database Syst Rev 2009;(4):CD006340. http://dx.doi.org/10.1002/14651858.CD006340.pub3.
39. Donohue FJ, Jain N. Exhaled nitric oxide to predict corticosteroid responsiveness and reduce asthma exacerbation rates. Respir Med 2013;107:943–52.
40. van der Valk RJ, Stern G, Freu U, et al. Daily exhaled nitric oxide measurement and asthma exacerbations in children. Allergy 2012;67:265–71.
41. Spencer AJ, Kahn RS, Hornung R, et al. Associations of fraction of exhaled nitric oxide with beta agonist use in children with asthma. Pediatr Allergy Immunol Pulmonol 2011;24:45–50.

Should Vitamin D Supplementation Be a Regular Part of Asthma Care?

Bruce R. Gordon, MA, MD[a,b,c],*

KEYWORDS

- Vitamin D • Vitamin D3 • Calcitriol • Calcidiol • Allergy • Asthma • Hypersensitivity
- Immunotherapy

KEY POINTS

- Vitamin D (vitD3) is important for immune system function.
- Low vitD3 may initiate asthma.
- VitD3 supplements may treat steroid-resistant asthma, reduce steroid-induced bone loss, improve immunotherapy (IT), decrease infections, and inhibit remodeling. Unfortunately, there are few adequate double-blind treatment studies.
- Calcidiol should be measured in every allergy patient. Accepted calcidiol serum values are less than 25 nmol/L (deficiency) and less than 50 to 72.5 nmol/L (insufficiency).
- VitD3 supplements up to 10,000 IU daily are safe. However, because of person-to-person variability in calcidiol levels produced by any supplement dose, calcidiol levels must be measured during treatment.
- Because it will be years until there is certainty about vitD3 benefits and optimum treatment levels, the decision to supplement depends on the severity of disease, history of infection and steroid use, IT status, and calcidiol level.

INTRODUCTION

There have been almost 400 scientific articles published on the relationship of vitamin D to allergic inflammation. Simultaneously, there has been growing clinical recognition that vitamin D deficiency occurs frequently in many patient populations. Therefore, the key questions clinical allergists must now ask are how do knowledge of vitamin D actions and the frequency of vitamin D deficiency influence clinical

Disclosures and conflicts of interest: The author has no financial relationship with any organization that might have an interest in this work, and there are no other relationships or activities that could influence, or seem to influence, this work.
[a] Cape Cod Hospital, 27 Park Street, Hyannis, MA 02601, USA; [b] Laryngology & Otology, Harvard University, 25 Shattuck Street, Boston, MA 02115, USA; [c] Massachusetts Eye & Ear Infirmary, 243 Charles Street, Boston, MA 02114, USA
* Cape Cod ENT, 65 Cedar Street, Hyannis, MA 02601.
E-mail address: docbruce@comcast.net

practice; should allergy patients be tested for vitamin D status; and, if deficient, should they receive vitamin D supplementation?

CALCITRIOL

The biologically most active form of vitamin D is calcitriol, 1,25-dihydroxy cholecalciferol (vitD3). A bioequivalent molecule, 1,25-dihydroxy ergocalciferol (vitamin D2), is formed from plant sterols. VitD3 is a steroid hormone acting via the nuclear vitamin D receptor (VDR) to activate or repress the expression of hundreds of genes that function in every tissue.[1] For example, calbindin, important in embryonic lung differentiation, is vitamin-D dependent.[2] Approximately 3% of all human genes are regulated by vitamin D, either solely or as a coregulator, often with vitamin A.[3] Secosteroids in food, found primarily in fish oil, artificially fortified foods, and, to a lesser extent, in plants, are first 25-hydroxylated by the liver to produce calcidiol, and then acted on by the kidney, antigen processing cells, lung epithelial cells, and other cell types, including almost all immune system cells.[4,5] This second hydroxylation, catalyzed by 1-α-hydroxylase, is the rate-limiting step in vitD3 synthesis, and is tightly controlled by a complex web of feedback loops.[5]

VitD3 can also be synthesized in skin from cholesterol, via photolysis by ultraviolet light. Long ago, sunlight was known to be important for health because of the obvious variation in rickets incidence and in infectious diseases with increased sunlight.[3,6] Importantly, the indoor existence of many people today easily can lead to vitamin D deficiency.[7] Institutionalized or hospital inpatients, poorly nourished individuals, and people living closer to the poles are at risk for vitamin D deficiency, as are persons of low socioeconomic status, elders, dark-skinned people, patients with cystic fibrosis or other chronic pulmonary diseases (including asthma), and tobacco users.[8] Cannell and colleagues,[9] and Pearce and Cheetham,[10] believe that most of the population in temperate zone countries now has vitamin D deficiency. Deficiency also commonly occurs in the Middle East and the tropics.[11,12] Despite these opinions, there are still so few long-term, randomized, vitamin D studies, that the Institute of Medicine (IOM) stated that current evidence indicates only about 2.5% of the North American population is actually vitamin D deficient.[13] The IOM report has been criticized as being overly conservative.[14] A comprehensive review of vitamin D studies has been done,[15] as well as a review of the impact of nutrition on asthma development.[16]

ILLNESSES ASSOCIATED WITH CALCITRIOL DEFICIENCY

The rare visible consequences of vitD3 deficiency are osteomalacia with fractures and pediatric rickets. Other potential consequences are less visible, including autoimmune illnesses, cancers, diabetes, metabolic syndrome, hypertension, infection susceptibility, adverse pregnancy outcomes, neurocognitive dysfunction, and a 26% higher all-causes mortality, all of which are associated with low vitamin D levels.[3,10,15] For example, a large data-mining study of unselected middle-aged people found that calcidiol levels less than 52.5 nmol/L were associated with significant increases in both cardiovascular and all-causes mortality.[17] The Third National Health and Nutrition Examination Survey (NHANES III) analyzed more than 14,000 adults and found a strong association between higher calcidiol levels and better pulmonary function.[8] Finally, one possible cause of the historic rise in asthma cases is vitamin D deficiency.[18] Low serum vitamin D levels are associated with poor asthma control, and low levels have been found to be common even in the Mediterranean region.[19] In the United States, a meta-analysis found 61% of young asthmatics have low serum calcidiol levels,[20] whereas 86% of young urban black asthmatics are calcitriol deficient, compared with 19% of nonasthmatic controls.[21] A final factor may be the recent rise in obesity because body fat content is inversely correlated with serum calcidiol level.[2]

MEASURING VITAMIN D

Serum vitD3 is fully bound by vitamin D binding protein (VDBP), which is present in great excess and has immunomodulatory properties independent of vitD3.[22] VDBP is secreted into the airway where it assists in macrophage activation, chemotaxis, and oxidative killing. Serum VDBP levels inversely correlate with lung function of patients with chronic obstructive pulmonary disease (COPD). VDBP levels are elevated in the airways of children with severe, poorly treated, unresponsive asthma; however, it is not known if this is cause or effect.[22]

Vitamin D status can be accurately determined by measuring calcidiol, 25-hydroxy cholecalciferol, in blood. There are two common measurement units for calcidiol, with a conversion factor of 1 ng/mL = 2.5 nmol/L. There is very active debate about the optimum serum calcidiol range, with the current consensus being 50 to 75 nmol/L,[23] or greater than 50 nmol/L.[13] However, based on observational studies, Grant[24] has proposed optimum levels of 75 to 100 nmol/L. According to the IOM, adequate calcidiol serum levels can normally be sustained by vitamin D supplements of 400 IU per day in infants, 600 IU per day for ages 1 to 70, and 800 IU per day over age 70.[13] However, in pregnancy, 4000 IU per day is required,[25] and some people may require supplements greater than 5000 IU per day.[9] See later discussion on supplementation.

VITAMIN D AFFECTS IMMUNE FUNCTION

The first evidence for immune effects of vitD3 was the 1983 discovery that human peripheral mononuclear cells and activated T-cells had VDRs,[26] and that vitD3 deficiency was a cause of delayed hypersensitivity anergy.[27] The following year, vitD3 was shown to be a stimulatory hormone for monocyte activation.[26,28] By 2004, vitD3 had been found to be an important selective immune system regulator, with complex effects that depend on the specific function being evaluated and on other environmental cofactors, especially calcium.[29] Both T-helper type (Th)1 and Th2 CD4+ cells increase their expression of VDR on activation. In addition, these cells respond to vitD3 by reducing proliferation and altering production of Th1 and Th2 cytokines.[29] The primary effects of vitD3 are to inhibit specific immunity; increase production of innate antimicrobial peptides, cathelicidin, and defensin β2; and promote the development and function of NK T-cells.[3] VitD3 is also essential for production of prohibitin, which regulates antioxidant defenses and apoptosis,[30] and for stimulation of antiinflammatory mast cells.[31] Most importantly, vitD3 inhibits the initiation of most Th1-mediated and Th2-mediated inflammatory diseases. A complicating finding is that there is evidence for different effects of vitD3 at different doses. Kuo and colleagues[18] studied both human peripheral monocytes and a monocyte-derived cell line in vitro. They found that vitD3 suppressed Th1 cytokines at low doses and stimulated Th2 cytokines at high doses.

VitD3 had long been known to affect macrophage, dendritic, and Th1 cells. However, it was not until 2004 that vitD3 effects on Th2 cells were found. Changes in Th2 cell migration and tissue homing led to reduced Th2 function at inflammation sites.[32] In a mouse VDR genetic knockout model (KO), compared with wild type (WT) mice, it was impossible to induce allergic asthma, implying a critical role for vitamin D in regulation of allergic inflammation.[33] These KO mice natively show a Th1 bias, which is normalized by vitD3 supplements,[29] and, experimental asthma can be induced in vitD3-treated KO mice just as successfully as in WT mice. Dietary vitD3 deficiency shifted the WT T-helper cell bias toward Th1, just as in the KO mice. These findings could indicate that vitD3 supplements would worsen allergic asthma. However, vitD3 supplementation of WT mice had no effect on either asthma induction or asthma severity.[29] On further analysis, the vitD3 receptor KO mice could develop peripheral Th2 inflammation, but, probably due to deceased cell trafficking, they did not develop lung inflammation.

GENETIC CONTROL OF VITAMIN D LEVELS AND THE RELATION TO ASTHMA

Human genome-wide linkage evaluation has shown strong genetic regulation of serum calcidiol levels, but not calcitriol levels.[34] Single nucleotide polymorphisms (SNPs) that reduce calcidiol levels usually affect activity of one of the two hydroxylases or the serum VDBP.[3] The second hydroxylation to active calcitriol is the rate-limiting step in synthesis. Production of the 1-hydroxylase is under extensive feedback control by cytokines and kinases that, by increasing vitD3 levels, help terminate ongoing immune inflammation. SNPs in genes for the 25-hydroxylase can directly affect presence of asthma, and SNPs in the VDR gene affect asthma morbidity and lung function, as well as number of positive allergen tests and IgE elevation.[35]

CONCOMITANT EFFECTS OF VITAMIN D AND CALCIUM

VitD3 and calcium work together for normal homeostasis, including immune functioning. Because vitD3 is necessary for intestinal absorption of both calcium and phosphate, insufficient calcidiol has a multiplier effect. VDR KO mice develop rickets, osteomalacia, and secondary hyperparathyroidism that are improved by calcium and phosphate supplementation.[36] In humans, calcium with vitD3 is effective in reducing hip fractures, unlike single supplements.[37] Dietary experiments with IL-10 KO mice that develop irritable bowel disease (IBD) show that combined calcium and vitD3 can completely prevent IBD, whereas supplements of only vitD3 or calcium are less effective.[29] Similar effects of calcium and vitD3 supplements were found in a mouse multiple sclerosis model. The IOM recommends daily calcium doses from 200 to 1300 mg, up to maximum daily doses of 1000 to 3000 mg, depending on age, sex, and pregnancy status.[13] The US Preventative Services Task Force recently reviewed the combined use of calcium and vitamin D supplements specifically for fracture prevention, and concluded that, although there is good evidence for an effect to prevent falls in all people over age 65, the evidence is inadequate to recommend supplement use for fracture prevention.[38]

In the past year, the cardiovascular safety of calcium supplements, but not calcium-containing foods, was questioned. A subsequent detailed reanalysis was done of the two epidemiologic studies and the meta-analysis that had raised concerns.[39] The review board found that there were sufficient problems with the methodology of those three studies and that many other good studies did not show elevated risks from calcium supplements. The board concluded that current calcium supplement guidelines should not be changed.

VITAMIN D EFFECTS ON ALLERGY AND ASTHMA

In vitro studies prove that vitD3 supplementation suppresses dendritic cell maturation and subsequent Th1 cell development by blocking IL-12 signaling.[40] Wjst[41] then proposed that infant vitD3 supplements, which had eliminated rickets, might actually be a reason for the rapid increase in allergy prevalence in developed countries. Wjst[41] cited several nutritional supplement studies as supporting data for a possible link between vitD3 supplementation and increased risk of food allergy sensitization, but acknowledged that there is still insufficient information to conclude how early vitD3 exposure affects the developing immune system. On the other hand, in adult mice with experimental asthma, prenatal vitD3 deficiency causes an increase in their allergic sensitized lymphocytes.[42]

One effect of vitD3 that could be relevant for asthma is the induction of innate natural killer (NK) T-cells and anti-infectious peptides.[4,31] In mice, inadequate vitD3 during embryogenesis causes a reduction in NK cells that cannot be remedied after birth.[43] Production of intracellular protective cathelicidins and defensin β2 is also vitD3 dependent.[31,44] In humans, naturally varying seasonal vitD3 levels have been found to inversely correlate with incidence of viral respiratory infections,[4,45] with calcidiol levels greater than 95 nmol/L being maximally protective. In children younger than age 5 in Hawaii, viral bronchiolitis, respiratory syncytial virus, and pneumonia vary with both season and skin pigmentation;[11] whereas, in England, monthly incidence of astrovirus and norovirus infections inversely correlates with calcidiol levels. Vitamin D treatment trials improved tuberculosis patients with VDR mutations[6] and substantially reduced winter viral infections in postmenopausal black women.[46]

Unlike the molecular and animal model data, which is complex and sometimes seems conflicting, most clinical observation studies show strong support for the idea that adequate vitamin D is a protective factor against asthma.[3] Luong and Nguyen,[2] and Gilbert and colleagues,[8] have reviewed vitD3 effects on asthma. In most human studies, vitD3 reduces the prevalence of asthma, prevents COPD, and does not aggravate allergic diseases.[3] VitD3 corrects, in vitro, the defective IL-10 secretion by CD4+ Treg cells from steroid-resistant asthma patients and makes these cells normally sensitive to steroids.[47] Calcidiol levels in many, but not all, studies are inversely correlated with asthma and wheezing incidences, in both children and adults, and are directly correlated with FEV1 values in asthma. Some studies also show an inverse correlation between calcidiol levels and IgE concentrations or eosinophil counts. Low calcidiol levels in pregnancy are associated with increased asthma and eczema in those children, and vitD3 supplementation of pregnant women reduces asthma risk in their children by 40%.[30] In another study, calcidiol cord blood levels did not predict the presence of asthma at age 5, even though both high and low calcidiol levels were associated with higher total and specific IgE levels.[48] A reason for the negative results of this one study may be the unknown intake of vitD3 during childhood, and that very few study infants had initially low calcidiol levels. Low calcidiol does predict greater risk of asthma-related hospitalization and increased use of asthma medication.[30] Finally, adequate vitamin D levels seem to protect asthmatic children from loss of bone calcium during treatment with oral corticosteroids.[49] If replicated, this single finding would make vitamin D supplementation essential in asthma care.

VITAMIN D EFFECTS ON IMMUNOTHERAPY AND TOLEROGENESIS

VitD3 may be effective as an adjuvant during immunotherapy (IT). In both mouse and human IT studies, vitD3 supplements have a suppressive effect on allergic inflammation, and offset the otherwise negative effects of oral corticosteroids on sublingual IT (SLIT) effectiveness in a mouse model[50] and in humans.[51] VitD3 pretreatment of adult mice, before sensitization, significantly enhances the effectiveness of allergy IT, and decreases both lung allergic inflammatory cells and cytokines.[52] In mice, vitD3 acts by stimulating dendritic cells, promoting development of both IL-10 producing and Foxp3+ Treg cells, thereby increasing tolerance.[50,53] These effects, unlike those produced by IT, are not antigen specific, so there is a potential benefit from using vitD3 in combination with IT. Corticosteroids were believed to have similar nonspecific effects on Treg development[53] and, when used together, corticosteroids and ViD3 might have enhancing effects on IT.[54] However, there was no human study of the effects of corticosteroids on IT. Majak and colleagues[54] tested these ideas by performing a three-arm, randomized, double-blind study in 48 asthmatic children, treated for a year with dust mite SLIT and prednisone 20 mg daily, plus or minus 1000 IU per week of vitD3 or placebo. Their key finding was that daily corticosteroids substantially decreased SLIT effectiveness and that vitamin D3 supplements prevented the deleterious effect of corticosteroids. This pilot study, along with effects of vitD3 on tolerogenesis (see later discussion), suggests that vitD3 supplements may help allergy IT efficacy.[51,54]

VitD3 inhibits the polarization of uncommitted T-cells to Th1 or Th2 and, instead, stimulates Treg production, leading to tolerogenesis.[3] Mouse cell cultures show vitD3 does so by directly suppressing transcription of interferon-γ and IL-10, respectively, the primary driving cytokines for Th1 and Th2 differentiation. One of the consequences of this tolerogenesis is that Th2 cells become relatively disinhibited compared with Th1 cells, which shifts the immune response to a Th2 bias. Unlike effects on Th1 and Th17 cells, which are clearly inhibitory,[55] studies of the effects of vitD3 on Th2 function are controversial, and show both inhibition and stimulation, depending on the experimental conditions. This in vitro enhancement of Treg function has now been confirmed to occur in asthmatic human airway lymphocytes, in which both Foxp3(+) and IL-10(+) Treg numbers are correlated with serum calcidiol levels.[56] Similar findings have been seen in human blood lymphocytes and this probably explains cases of asthma that do not respond to steroids.[57] It is likely that vitamin D-related Treg function has strong clinical significance for asthma development and control.

VITAMIN D EFFECTS ON INFLAMMATION AND BRONCHIAL REMODELING

Perhaps the most significant effect of vitD3 on asthma is a strong, direct antiinflammatory effect, evident from the suppression of both bronchial smooth muscle proliferation, and mucus and matrix metalloproteinase secretion by cultured human bronchial cells.[58] VitD3 treatment also increases smooth muscle cell vitamin D receptors and, at physiologic concentrations, partially prevents smooth muscle cells from becoming passively sensitized by exposure to asthmatic serum.[58] Similarly, in rats, vitD3 treatment, either before or after allergic sensitization, significantly reduced acute asthma. VitD3 effects on acute asthma were comparable to corticosteroid treatment. It reduced chronic asthma by decreasing both exhaled nitric oxide and induced nitric oxide synthetase.[59] Finally, in human airway smooth muscle cells, vitD3 inhibits secretion of the eosinophil chemoattractant, RANTES.[4] These observations raise hope that vitD3 supplements could have benefit in asthma treatment because eosinophil influx, smooth muscle cell proliferation, matrix metalloproteinase production, and induction of nitric oxide synthetase are primary elements of remodeling and subsequent development of chronic bronchial hyper-reactivity and loss of lung function.[60]

EVIDENCE OF SAFETY AND EFFICACY OF VITAMIN D SUPPLEMENTS

If vitD3 supplementation is to be useful, it is important to know how best to administer vitamin D supplements, the optimum serum level, and the level at which toxicity may occur. The most recent reviews of this subject conclude that, although there is substantial observational evidence for beneficial effects of vitD3 supplementation on many disorders, there is a lack of adequate double-blind studies. Some studies also show a J-shaped or U-shaped dose-effect curve, which implies there might be adverse effects of vitD3 at high doses.[13,23,61] On the other hand, compliance is poor with daily dosing, and some people require surprisingly high doses of vitD3 (over 4000 IU/day) to achieve adequate serum levels, which encouraged intermittent high-dose treatment. This may not be the right approach, as indicated by two studies of annual high dose vitD3 pulse dosing that show an increase in both falls and in fractures, the opposite from the expected effect. Lower doses at shorter intervals, such as every 4 months, have not shown any increase in fractures, so it is likely that large, infrequent swings in vitD3 levels are deleterious.[23]

A second area that must be addressed is the lack of agreement by experts on what should be considered a normal serum calcidiol level. Although 10 ng/mL (25 nmol/L) of calcidiol has been generally accepted for years as the threshold for severe vitamin D deficiency, the upper level for insufficiency now seems to be at least 50 to 75 nmol/L.[23] The bulk of current evidence from biochemical and observational data, and from a few randomized trials, supports calcidiol serum levels of at least 50 nmol/L to normalize serum parathyroid hormone levels, minimize risk of osteomalacia, and provide optimum bone and muscle function. Higher levels of vitD3, in the presence of adequate calcium, do not further increase musculoskeletal health. However, observational studies show that nonskeletal systems may require calcidiol levels greater than 70 to 80 nmol/L to maximally decrease certain cancers (especially colon, breast, ovarian, and prostate), mental disorders, autoimmunity, infections, and cardiovascular diseases.[23] For example, a meta-analysis of vitD3-related mortality studies found progressively lower mortality with increasing calcidiol levels up to 87.5 nmol/L.[62] The 2011 Endocrine Society Clinical Practice Guideline (ESCPG) gives consensus values for vitamin D deficiency as calcidiol serum levels less than 50 nmol/liter, and vitamin D insufficiency as calcidiol serum levels of 52.5 to 72.5 nmol/liter.[63] It is unlikely that there will be a universally accepted desirable calcidiol dose range until very long-term vitamin D supplementation trials that monitor all of the illnesses noted above are done in humans.

A third concern is possible toxicity of vitD3, from hypercalcemia, hypercalciuria, and possible renal calculi or tissue calcification. These complications are very rare and, fortunately, a range of possible calcidiol serum levels and oral doses has been found to be safe. The results of toxicity studies include:

- Sanders and colleagues[23] state that no toxicity has been observed below calcidiol levels of 220 nmol/L, and only occasional toxicity occurs up to 500 nmol/L.
- Grant[64] believes that there is no reliable evidence for adverse health effects of calcidiol in the range of 75 to 125 nmol/L. Based on a 6-month study,[65] daily 4000 IU of vitD3 is safe and usually raises calcidiol levels to about 140 nmol/L.
- Another study showed no toxicity after 5 months of 10,000 IU daily.[8]
- Another study showed 4000 IU vitD3 supplements beginning at about 14 weeks, and continued throughout pregnancy, is safe.[25]
- The IOM, for age 9 and older, recommends up to 4000 IU/day as safe.[13]
- The 2011 ESCPG lists age-based treatment guidelines for persons found to be vitD3 deficient.[63] For adults, they recommend weekly 50,000 IU of vitD3 for 8 weeks, or daily vitD3, to achieve a calcidiol level above 75 nmol/L, followed by maintenance treatment of 1500 to 2000 IU per day. For obese patients or persons with malabsorption, they recommend 6000 to 10,000 IU per day for treatment, followed by maintenance of 3000 to 6000 IU per day.

The results of any of these vitD3 doses must be checked by actual serum calcidiol measurements (see later discussion).

A final concern is how the variability of individuals affects supplementation. Garland and colleagues[66] repeatedly measured calcidiol levels in over 3500 unselected, health-conscious adults, and compared their serum levels with their reported use of vitamin D supplements. The estimated mean daily vitamin D input (as food and sun exposure, not due to supplements) was a surprising 3300 IU daily. Both for men and women, supplement doses of vitamin D up to 10,000 IU per day did not produce serum calcidiol levels greater than 200 ng/mL, at which toxicity might occur. Only at 50,000 IU per day did even a few people develop levels from 200 to 250 ng/mL. At all supplement doses, about a sixfold person-to-person variation was seen in the serum calcidiol level achieved by any particular dose. Because the relationship of supplement dose to serum calcidiol level is not linear, but a flattening curve, it takes larger dose increments to raise high calcidiol levels still higher. Other treatment trials have also noted substantial variability in serum calcitriol levels achieved with any single vitD3 dose. These facts indicate that, during treatment or maintenance supplementation, measurement of serum calcidiol levels is critically important to ensure that the treatment goal is actually achieved.

SUMMARY

It is clear from molecular and animal model research that vitD3 performs critically important functions in virtually every body tissue, including almost all immune system cells. The general effect of higher vitD3 levels is immune suppression of the adaptive response by induced tolerance and production of a relative Th2 bias, with the important exception that NK cells and antimicrobial peptides are stimulated. The overall balance of tolerance and stimulation in any individual depends on many factors and probably includes vitD3 levels during embryogenesis, as well as later in life. Many human observation studies show strong associations between low vitD3 levels and development of important diseases in which a Th1 or Th2 inflammatory response is believed to play a role, such as autoimmune illnesses, cancers, diabetes, cardiovascular disease, infectious diseases, asthma, and all-causes mortality. Whether vitD3 supplements could reduce the risk of developing these diseases, or ameliorate them, remains unknown. Some reports also suggest that vitD3 could be useful for treating steroid-resistant asthma, preventing bone loss during oral steroid therapy, improving IT results, and decreasing viral winter infections. VitD3 may also inhibit lung remodeling and bronchial reactivity, and potentially improve pulmonary function. However, few double-blind vitD3 supplementation studies have been done, so that none of these observations is solidly proven. Authorities disagree on optimal serum vitD3 levels, but the most commonly accepted values are less than 25 nmol/L for deficiency and less than 50 to 72.5 nmol/L for insufficiency. Over-the-counter daily vitD3 supplements up to 10,000 IU have a wide safety margin but, because of substantial person-to-person variability in calcidiol levels produced by a given supplement dose, blood levels must be measured during treatment. It will likely be many years until we have certainty about the benefits and know optimum treatment levels for vitD3 supplements.

Ultimately, the decision to supplement or not with vitD3 is a clinical decision made with each allergy patient after considering the severity of their disease, infection and steroid use history, IT status, and their calcidiol level. The only certainty is that every allergy patient should have their calcidiol level measured, to ensure that undetected vitD3 deficiency is not exacerbating their allergic disease, making IT less effective, or contributing to infectious exacerbations of their rhinitis or asthma.

ACKNOWLEDGMENTS

The author thanks the staff from Frazier-Grant Medical Library, Cape Cod Hospital, for expert research assistance: Jeanie Vander Pyl, MLIS, library director, June Bianchi, library assistant, and Deborah Tustin, MLIS, library assistant. Richard L. Mabry, MD and William M. Gordon, PhD provided editorial assistance.

REFERENCES

1. Pike JW. Genome-wide principles of gene regulation by the vitamin D receptor and its activating ligand. Mol Cell Endocrinol 2011;347(1–2):3–10.
2. Luong KV, Nguyen LT. The role of vitamin D in asthma. Pulm Pharmacol Ther 2012;25(2):137–43.
3. Székely JI, Pataki Á. Effects of vitamin D on immune disorders with special regard to asthma, COPD and autoimmune diseases: a short review. Expert Rev Respir Med 2012;6(6):683–704.
4. Sandhu MS, Casale TB. The role of vitamin D in asthma. Ann Allergy Asthma Immunol 2010;105(3):191–9.
5. Baeke F, Takiishi T, Korf H, et al. Vitamin D: modulator of the immune system. Curr Opin Pharmacol 2010;10(4):482–96.
6. Wolden-Kirk H, Gysemans C, Verstuyf A, et al. Extraskeletal effects of vitamin D. Endocrinol Metab Clin North Am 2012;41:571–94.
7. Godar DE, Pope SJ, Grant WB, et al. Solar UV doses of adult Americans and vitamin D(3) production. Dermatoendocrinol 2011;3(4):243–50.
8. Gilbert CR, Arum SM, Smith CM. Vitamin D deficiency and chronic lung disease. Can Respir J 2009;16(3):75–80.
9. Cannell JJ, Hollis BW, Zasloff M, et al. Diagnosis and treatment of vitamin D deficiency. Expert Opin Pharmacother 2008;9(1):107–18.
10. Pearce SH, Cheetham TD. Diagnosis and management of vitamin D deficiency. BMJ 2010;340:b5664.
11. Grant WB. Variations in vitamin D production could possibly explain the seasonality of childhood respiratory infections in Hawaii. Pediatr Infect Dis J 2008;27:853.
12. Al Anouti F, Thomas J, Abdel-Wareth L, et al. Vitamin D deficiency and sun avoidance among university students at Abu Dhabi, United Arab Emirates. Dermatoendocrinol 2011;3(4):235–9.
13. Ross AC, Manson JE, Abrams SA, et al. The 2011 report on dietary reference intakes for calcium and vitamin D from the Institute of Medicine: what clinicians need to know. J Clin Endocrinol Metab 2011;96(1):53–8.
14. Grant WB, Tangpricha V. Vitamin D: its role in disease prevention. Dermatoendocrinol 2012;4(2):81–3.
15. Pludowski P, Holick MF, Pilz S, et al. Vitamin D effects on musculoskeletal health, immunity, autoimmunity, cardiovascular disease, cancer, fertility, pregnancy, dementia and mortality—A review of recent evidence. Autoimmun Rev 2013. Available at: http://dx.doi.org/10.1016/j.autrev.2013.02.004.
16. Allan K, Devereux G. Diet and asthma: nutrition implications from prevention to treatment. J Am Diet Assoc 2011;111(2):258–68.
17. Amer M, Qayyum R. Relationship between 25-hydroxyvitamin D and all-cause and cardiovascular disease mortality. Am J Med 2013;126(6):509–14.
18. Kuo YT, Kuo CH, Lam KP, et al. Effects of vitamin D3 on expression of tumor necrosis factor-alpha and chemokines by monocytes. J Food Sci 2010;75(6):H200–4.

19. Chinellato I, Piazza M, Sandri M, et al. Vitamin D serum levels and markers of asthma control in Italian children. J Pediatr 2011;158(3):437–41.

20. Paul G, Brehm JM, Alcorn JF, et al. Vitamin D and asthma. Am J Respir Crit Care Med 2012;185(2):124–32.

21. Freishtat RJ, Iqbal SF, Pillai DK, et al. High prevalence of vitamin D deficiency among inner-city African American youth with asthma in Washington, DC. J Pediatr 2010;156(6):948–52.

22. Gupta A, Dimeloe S, Richards DF, et al. Vitamin D binding protein and asthma severity in children. J Allergy Clin Immunol 2012;129(6):1669–71.

23. Sanders KM, Nicholson GC, Ebeling PR. Is high dose vitamin D harmful? Calcif Tissue Int 2013;92:191–206, 491–2.

24. Grant WB. Re: key questions in vitamin D research. Scand J Clin Lab Invest 2013;73(2):182–3.

25. Hollis BW, Johnson D, Hulsey TC, et al. Vitamin D supplementation during pregnancy: double-blind, randomized clinical trial of safety and effectiveness. J Bone Miner Res 2011;26(10):2341–57.

26. Bhalla AK, Amento EP, Clemens TL, et al. Specific high-affinity receptors for 1,25-dihydroxyvitamin D3 in human peripheral blood mononuclear cells: presence in monocytes and induction in T lymphocytes following activation. J Clin Endocrinol Metab 1983;57(6):1308–10.

27. Toss G, Symreng T. Delayed hypersensitivity response and vitamin D deficiency. Int J Vitam Nutr Res 1983;53(1):27–31.

28. Amento EP, Bhalla AK, Kurnick JT, et al. 1 alpha, 25-dihydroxyvitamin D3 induces maturation of the human monocyte cell line U937, and, in association with a factor from human T lymphocytes, augments production of the monokine, mononuclear cell factor. J Clin Invest 1984;73(3):731–9.

29. Cantorna MT, Zhu Y, Froicu M, et al. Vitamin D status, 1,25-dihydroxyvitamin D3, and the immune system. Am J Clin Nutr 2004;80(Suppl 6):1717S–20S.

30. Agrawal T, Gupta GK, Agrawal DK. Vitamin D deficiency decreases the expression of VDR and prohibitin in the lungs of mice with allergic airway inflammation. Exp Mol Pathol 2012;93(1):74–81.

31. Youssef DA, Miller CW, El-Abbassi AM, et al. Antimicrobial implications of vitamin D. Dermatoendocrinol 2011;3(4):220–9.

32. Topilski I, Flaishon L, Naveh Y, et al. The anti-inflammatory effects of 1,25-dihydroxyvitamin D3 on Th2 cells in vivo are due in part to the control of integrin-mediated T lymphocyte homing. Eur J Immunol 2004;34(4):1068–76.

33. Wittke A, Weaver V, Mahon BD, et al. Vitamin D receptor-deficient mice fail to develop experimental allergic asthma. J Immunol 2004;173(5):3432–6.

34. Wjst M, Altmüller J, Faus-Kessler T, et al. Asthma families show transmission disequilibrium of gene variants in the vitamin D metabolism and signaling pathway. Respir Res 2006;7(60):1–11.

35. Pillai DK, Iqbal SF, Benton AS, et al. Associations between genetic variants in vitamin D metabolism and asthma characteristics in young African Americans: a pilot study. J Investig Med 2011;59(6):938–46.

36. Christakos S, DeLuca HF. Minireview: vitamin D: is there a role in extraskeletal health? Endocrinology 2011;152(8):2930–6.

37. Murad MH, Drake MT, Mullan RJ, et al. Clinical review. Comparative effectiveness of drug treatments to prevent fragility fractures: a systematic review and network meta-analysis. J Clin Endocrinol Metab 2012;97(6):1871–80.

38. Moyer VA. Vitamin D and calcium supplementation to prevent fractures in adults: U.S. Preventive Services Task Force Recommendation Statement. Ann Intern Med 2013;158:691–6.

39. Heaney RP, Kopecky S, Maki KC, et al. A review of calcium supplements and cardiovascular disease risk. Adv Nutr 2012;3(6):763–71.

40. Pedersen AW, Claesson MH, Zocca MB. Dendritic cells modified by vitamin D: future immunotherapy for autoimmune diseases. Vitam Horm 2011;86:63–82.

41. Wjst M. The vitamin D slant on allergy. Pediatr Allergy Immunol 2006;17(7):477–83.

42. Gorman S, Tan DH, Lambert MJ, et al. Vitamin D3 deficiency enhances allergen-induced lymphocyte responses in a mouse model of allergic airway disease. Pediatr Allergy Immunol 2012;23:83–7.

43. Cantorna MT, Zhao J, Yang L. Vitamin D, invariant natural killer T-cells and experimental autoimmune disease. Proc Nutr Soc 2012;71(1):62–6.

44. White JH. Vitamin D as an inducer of cathelicidin antimicrobial peptide expression: past, present and future. J Steroid Biochem Mol Biol 2010;121(1–2):234–8.

45. Sabetta JR, DePetrillo P, Cipriani RJ, et al. Serum 25-hydroxyvitamin D and the incidence of acute viral respiratory tract infections in healthy adults. PLoS One 2010;5(6):e11088.

46. Aloia JF, Li-Ng M. Epidemic influenza and vitamin D. Epidermol Infect 2007;135: 1095–6.

47. Xystrakis E, Kusumakar S, Boswell S, et al. Reversing the defective induction of IL-10-secreting regulatory T-cells in glucocorticoid-resistant asthma patients. J Clin Invest 2006;116(1):146–55.

48. Rothers J, Wright AL, Stern DA, et al. Cord blood 25-hydroxyvitamin D levels are associated with aeroallergen sensitization in children from Tucson, Arizona. J Allergy Clin Immunol 2011;128(5):1093–9.

49. Tse SM, Kelly HW, Litonjua AA, et al. Corticosteroid use and bone mineral accretion in children with asthma: effect modification by vitamin D. J Allergy Clin Immunol 2012;130:53–60.

50. Van Overtvelt L, Lombardi V, Razafindratsita A, et al. IL-10-inducing adjuvants enhance sublingual immunotherapy efficacy in a murine asthma model. Int Arch Allergy Immunol 2008;145(2):152–62.

51. van Hemelen D, van Oosterhout AJ. Adjuvants for immunotherapy: lost in translation? Clin Exp Allergy 2009;39(12):1783–5.

52. Ma JX, Xia JB, Cheng XM, et al. 1,25-dihydroxyvitamin D_3 pretreatment enhances the efficacy of allergen immunotherapy in a mouse allergic asthma model. Chin Med J (Engl) 2010;123(24):3591–6.

53. Robinson DS. Regulatory T-cells and asthma. Clin Exp Allergy 2009;39(9): 1314–23.

54. Majak P, Rychlik B, Stelmach I. The effect of oral steroids with and without vitamin D3 on early efficacy of immunotherapy in asthmatic children. Clin Exp Allergy 2009;39(12):1830–41.

55. Bansal AS, Henriquez F, Sumar N, et al. T helper cell subsets in arthritis and the benefits of immunomodulation by $1,25(OH)_2$ vitamin D. Rheumatol Int 2012; 32(4):845–52.

56. Urry Z, Chambers ES, Xystrakis E, et al. The role of 1α,25-dihydroxyvitamin D3 and cytokines in the promotion of distinct Foxp3+ and IL-10+ CD4+ T-cells. Eur J Immunol 2012;42(10):2697–708.

57. Chambers ES, Nanzer AM, Richards DF, et al. Serum 25-dihydroxyvitamin D levels correlate with CD41 Foxp31 T-cell numbers in moderate/severe asthma. J Allergy Clin Immunol 2012;130(2):542–4.

58. Song Y, Qi H, Wu C. Effect of 1,25-(OH)2D3 (a vitamin D analogue) on passively sensitized human airway smooth muscle cells. Respirology 2007;12(4):486–94.
59. Zhou Y, Zhou X, Wang X. 1,25-Dihydroxyvitamin D3 prevented allergic asthma in a rat model by suppressing the expression of inducible nitric oxide synthase. Allergy Asthma Proc 2008;29(3):258–67.
60. Clifford RL, Knox AJ. Vitamin D-a new treatment for airway remodelling in asthma? Br J Pharmacol 2009;158(6):1426–8.
61. Chen LY, Zhou XJ, Li X, et al. Effect of 1,25-(OH)2D3 supplementation during gestation and lactation on TGF-β1 and Smad3 expression in lungs of rat offspring with asthma. Zhongguo Dang Dai Er Ke Za Zhi 2012;14(5):366–70.
62. Zittermann A, Iodice S, Pilz S, et al. Vitamin D deficiency and mortality risk in the general population: a meta-analysis of prospective cohort studies. Am J Clin Nutr 2012;95(1):91–100.
63. Holick MF, Binkley NC, Bischoff-Ferrari HA, et al. Evaluation, treatment, and prevention of vitamin D deficiency: an Endocrine Society Clinical Practice Guideline. J Clin Endocrinol Metab 2011;96(7):1911–30.
64. Grant WB. Re: is high dose vitamin D harmful? Calcif Tissue Int 2013;92:489–90.
65. Vieth R, Chan P, MacFarlane G. Efficacy and safety of vitamin D3 input exceeding the lowest observed adverse effect concentration. Am J Clin Nutr 2001;73:288–94.
66. Garland CF, French CB, Baggerly LL, et al. Vitamin D supplement doses and serum 25-hydroxyvitamin D in the range associated with cancer prevention. Anticancer Res 2011;31:617–22.

Identifying Asthma Triggers

Justin C. McCarty, BA[a], Berrylin J. Ferguson, MD[b],*

KEYWORDS

- Reflux • Paradoxic vocal fold dysfunction • Obesity • Asthma triggers • Sinusitis
- Inhalant allergies • Food allergies

KEY POINTS

- Asthma may have one or many triggers.
- Identification and management of the trigger improves management.
- Common triggers include inhalants (allergens or irritants); food allergies (IgE and non-IgE mediated); gastroesophageal reflux; cyclooxygenase 1 inhibitors, such as aspirin in aspirin-exacerbated respiratory disease; and rhinosinusitis.
- Mimics of asthma include paradoxic vocal fold dysfunction.
- Comorbidities that exacerbate asthma include obesity.

INTRODUCTION

In medicine, the maxim that an ounce of prevention is worth a pound of cure plays a pivotal role in efficacious and cost-effective patient care. Asthma, with its pathogenesis rooted in atopy and airway hyperresponsiveness, can be treated in part by knowledge of and subsequent avoidance of the various triggers. Although asthma is associated with an allergic diathesis, an allergic trigger is only true or partly true in a subset of patients. This article reviews familiar allergic triggers and their management, and comorbid associations that worsen asthma or even mimic asthma without true bronchial hyperresponsiveness. In many patients there is more than one factor or trigger for the asthma, and optimal control is obtained when the patient and health care team work together to prevent exposure or ameliorate the aggravating condition, such as environmental allergens (pollen, dust mites, pet dander, and mold in the allergic patient with asthma). Other triggers or mimics of asthma symptoms are laryngopharyngeal reflux (LPR), also known as gastroesophageal reflux disease (GERD); exercise; irritants (tobacco smoke and industrial pollutants); food allergies; viral infections; pharmacologic agents (aspirin and β-blockers); and paradoxic vocal fold dysfunction (PVFD). Associations under investigation include obesity, stress, and hormonal status.

[a] Lake Erie of Osteopathic Medicine, 5000 Lakewood Ranch Boulevard, Bradenton, FL 34211–4909, USA; [b] UPMC Mercy, University of Pittsburgh School of Medicine, 1400 Locust Street, Suite B11500, Pittsburgh, PA 15219, USA
* Corresponding author.
E-mail address: fergusonbj@upmc.edu

Otolaryngol Clin N Am 47 (2014) 109–118
http://dx.doi.org/10.1016/j.otc.2013.08.012
0030-6665/14/$ – see front matter © 2014 Elsevier Inc. All rights reserved.

INHALANT TRIGGERS

The initial assessment of a patient should follow a systematic series of questions to identify possible exacerbating factors (**Fig. 1**). Once preliminarily identified, specific triggers then elicit an appropriate algorithm of inquiry. It is necessary to identify the precipitating factors to optimally direct therapy or avoidance. When evaluating irritant

Inhalant allergens
Does the patient have symptoms year round? (If yes, ask the following questions. If no, see next set of questions).
Does the patient keep pets indoors? What type?
Does the patient have moisture or dampness in any room of his or her home (eg, basement)? (Suggests house dust mites, molds).
Does the patient have mold visible in any part of his or her home? (Suggests molds).
Has the patient seen cockroaches or rodents in his or her home in the past month? (Suggests significant exposure).
Assume exposure to house dust mites unless patient lives in a semiarid region. However, if a patient living in a semiarid region uses a swamp cooler, exposure to house dust mites must still be assumed.
Do symptoms get worse at certain times of the year? (If yes, ask when symptoms occur).
Early spring? (Trees).
Late spring? (Grasses).
Late summer to autumn? (Weeds).
Summer and fall? (Alternaria, Cladosporium, mites).
Cold months in temperate climates? (Animal dander).

Tobacco smoke
Does the patient smoke?
Does anyone smoke at home or work?
Does anyone smoke at the child's daycare?

Indoor/outdoor pollutants and irritants
Is a wood-burning stove or fireplace used in the patient's home?
Are there unvented stoves or heaters in the patient's home?
Does the patient have contact with other smells or fumes from perfumes, cleaning agents, or sprays?
Have there been recent renovations or painting in the home?

Workplace exposures
Does the patient cough or wheeze during the week, but not on weekends when away from work?
Do the patient's eyes and nasal passages get irritated soon after arriving at work?
Do coworkers have similar symptoms?
What substances are used in the patient's worksite? (Assess for sensitizers).

Rhinitis
Does the patient have constant or seasonal nasal congestion, runny nose, and/or postnasal drip?

Gastroesophageal reflux disease (GERD)
Does the patient have heartburn?
Does food sometimes come up into the patient's throat?
Has the patient had coughing, wheezing, or shortness of breath at night in the past four weeks?
Does the infant vomit, followed by cough, or have wheezy cough at night? Are symptoms worse after feeding?

Sulfite sensitivity
Does the patient have wheezing, coughing, or shortness of breath after eating shrimp, dried fruit, or processed potatoes or after drinking beer or wine?

Medication sensitivities and contraindications
What medications does the patient use now (prescription and nonprescription)?
Does the patient use eyedrops? What type?
Does the patient use any medications that contain beta-blockers?
Does the patient ever take aspirin or other nonsteroidal antiinflammatory drugs?
Has the patient ever had symptoms of asthma after taking any of these medications?

Fig. 1. Assessment questions for environmental and other factors that can make asthma worse. These questions are examples and do not represent a standardized assessment or diagnostic instrument. The validity and reliability of these questions have not been assessed. (*From* National Heart, Blood, and Lung Institute. Expert panel report 3 (EPR 3): guidelines for the diagnosis and management of asthma. NIH Publication no. 08-4051.)

or allergic exposures as triggers, include the amount of exposure; patient sensitivity to a specific allergen; place of exposure to the asthma trigger (home, work, school); and clinical significance of sensitivity in how it relates to the patient's medical history.[1]

Unlike environmental allergens, in which the clinician is in part guided by allergy test results, such irritants as workplace chemicals and cigarette smoke trigger asthma through non–IgE mediated mechanisms and it can often be difficult to definitively identify the culprit, beyond the fact that the patient develops symptoms on entering the workplace, which are relieved when at home or in another environment. Formaldehyde outgassing of new construction and carpets can also trigger symptoms in poorly ventilated areas in some patients and reaches particularly high levels in mobile homes.[2] Glutaraldehyde, commonly used as a disinfectant for endoscopes, can be a trigger in the workplace.[3]

INHALANT ALLERGY

Allergens play a key role in many patients' allergies as a trigger of acute exacerbations and as underlying long-term effects on control. Allergens activation of mast cells with bound IgE leads to the release of bronchoconstrictor mediators, which results in the bronchial narrowing that characterizes asthma and symptoms of allergic rhinitis.[4] The most common allergen triggers, with slight differences in their effects, include *Dermatophagoides* species (dust mites), which cause perennial low-grade chronic symptoms; domestic animals (cats, dogs, cockroaches) causing perennial symptoms; and grass, ragweed, tree pollen, and fungal spores, which are seasonal but more often cause allergic rhinitis rather than asthma symptoms.[1] Environmental factors, such as thunderstorms, can increase the amount of pollen in the air attributed to conditions at the beginning of the storm causing pollen grains to rupture and disperse into the air.[5]

Recommendations that can be applied generally to allergens as an asthma trigger follow a systematic approach. After identification of the allergen, the environmental controls range from the simple to the complex. If water damage exists in the patient's dwelling and the patient is reactive to mold, then correction of the water leak and damage and remediation of any mold is requisite to improving the patient's health. This can be quite expensive. However, if dust mite or cockroach is a trigger, then pillow and mattress allergen covers coupled with hot water weekly washings of bed coverings may suffice in the former, and a visit from a pest control company on a scheduled basis may resolve the latter. Except in the most obvious cases, allergy skin or in vitro testing for IgE to specific antigens is the best way to identify potential allergens. Not every positive test represents a clinically important allergen. For example, in the 2005 NHANES study, more than 50% of the population demonstrated skin allergy test positivity to dust mite, whereas only about 20% of the population is allergic.[6] Similarly, up to 30% of allergens noted clinically by patients and negative on skin testing are positive on nasal provocation or assessment of nasal-specific IgE to the allergen.

If complete avoidance is not possible, then limiting exposure should be attempted. If there is no way to completely avoid or limit exposure, then a third option is for the patient to take an extra dose of bronchodilator and antihistamine before predicted trigger exposure or to undergo desensitization therapy either with allergy shots or sublingual drops.[1]

VIRAL TRIGGERS

One of the most common triggers of acute exacerbation is an upper respiratory tract infection, such as rhinovirus, respiratory syncytial virus, or coronavirus.[4] These viral infections, by poorly understood mechanisms, result in an increase in the numbers of eosinophils and neutrophils. People with asthma additionally may have reduced production of type 1 interferons by respiratory epithelial cells, thus increasing their susceptibility to viral infections and resulting in a greater inflammatory response when infection does occur. Patients may present with infections including colds, influenza, respiratory syncytial virus, and airway inflammation with concomitant increased mucus production. In patients with asthma, a viral infection can exacerbate inflammation that persists long after the viral part of the infection has resolved. Viral infections may also increase patient susceptibility to developing new allergic sensitivities.[7]

Patient recommendations to avoid infection follow advice that is applicable to all patients but that is especially important for people with asthma. Patients should be informed of the importance of washing their hands; avoiding sick contacts; getting adequate sleep; and using their prescribed medications for symptomatic treatment of the infection (intranasal glucocorticoids, decongestants).[8] It is recommended that people with asthma get yearly intramuscular flu vaccines; and there is evidence that people with asthma and others with chronic obstructive pulmonary disease may benefit from pneumococcal vaccine because of reductions in morbidity and mortality in these groups.[9,10]

GERD OR LPR

GERD or LPR is a commonly encountered comorbidity seen in people with asthma.[11,12] In one review of 28 studies GERD symptoms were seen in 59%, abnormal 24-hour pH tests in 51%, hiatal hernia in 51%, and esophagitis in 37%.[13] The symptoms of LPR include heartburn; regurgitation; dysphagia; chest pain; hoarseness; dental erosions; worsening in supine position; and worsening with such factors as eating, alcohol, theophylline, and systemic β-adrenergic agonists. Bronchodilators lower esophageal sphincter tone. Acid reflux may cause bronchoconstriction by three proposed mechanisms: (1) increased vagal tone, (2) sensitization of bronchial reactivity, and (3) microaspiration of gastric contents in the upper airway.[14–17]

Patient recommendations about the significance of LPR control and asthma symptoms have been variable in their outcomes in various trials. The recommendations can be split into two groups: patients with symptomatic LPR and patients that are asymptomatic. Patients with symptomatic LPR may benefit from a proton pump inhibitor (PPI) primarily in patients' subjective criteria based on studies quality of life questionnaires and in reducing the number of asthma exacerbations.[18] The studies that show improvement in pulmonary function in patients with asthma with GERD controlled with PPI showed only minor improvements.[19] In patients with asthma with clinically silent LPR, PPI therapy has not been shown to be of benefit in asthma outcomes, and it can be concluded that in these situations difficult-to-control asthma is not likely from GERD.[20,21] The approach should be to identify those patients most likely to benefit from PPI therapy, which are those with symptoms of regurgitation, nocturnal asthma, and most importantly concurrent symptoms of LPR and asthma. Patients should additionally follow the recommendations given to all patients with LPR, which include raising the head of the bed at night by 6 to 8 inches; not eating 2 to 3 hours before lying in supine position; avoiding fatty foods, chocolate, peppermint, and excessive alcohol; and reduction of abdominal obesity.[22] If clinical suspicion for LPR is high, then a trial of PPIs can be given. If the patient does not improve clinically, then further testing can be undertaken, such as 24-hour esophageal pH testing to help determine the cause.[23]

MEDICATION TRIGGERS AND ASPIRIN-EXACERBATED RESPIRATORY DISEASE

The most important medications to be aware of as triggering reactive airway are nonselective β-blockers, aspirin, and other nonsteroidal anti-inflammatory drugs

(NSAIDs). Although potentially nonselective β-blockers are contraindicated in all people with asthma, only about 5% of those with asthma or up to 40% of people with asthma with nasal polyps are triggered by aspirin or NSAIDs. These patients are classified as having aspirin-exacerbated respiratory disease (AERD), which is also commonly known as Samter triad: asthma, aspirin sensitivity, and nasal polyps.[24–27] Reactions to NSAIDs in those with AERD are classified as pseudoallergic because it is not a typical IgE-mediated reaction but rather is based on the common ability of NSAIDs and aspirin to inhibit the cyclooxygenase (COX)-1 enzyme. The pathophysiology of AERD is incompletely understood and most likely is related to overproduction of proinflammatory arachiadonic acid products, especially the leukotrienes. This is supported by the fact that medications that inhibit leukotriene synthesis and leukotriene receptor antagonists (eg, zileuton, montelukast) reduce or eliminate the bronchoconstrictive response to aspirin.[28–30] The diagnosis of AERD is based initially on clinical features being present. If Samter triad is present, the diagnosis can be relatively unambiguous, but more often only part of the triad is present or each part develops slowly over time making the association more difficult.[31] When suspicion of NSAID reaction is aroused, the physician should question the patient about any NSAID use after the first suspected reaction and whether any reaction occurred at that point, the reason being that NSAID sensitivity is acquired and thus prior nonreactivity is not as relevant.[26] Aspirin challenge is the only way to definitively diagnose NSAID sensitivity. There is an 80% likelihood of positive oral aspirin challenge with a history of a single NSAID reaction, which increases to 90% with history of two reactions.[32] Aspirin challenge is only needed in cases where a patient has ongoing regular need for NSAID therapy, such as rheumatologic disease or cardiovascular disease. These patients should be referred to an allergy or pulmonary specialist for the test.

Patient recommendations in AERD include typical asthma therapy with avoidance of all COX-1–inhibiting NSAIDs or aspirin desensitization followed by daily aspirin therapy. Pharmacologic therapy should include a leukotriene modifying agent, which can result in better asthma control than medium to high doses of glucocorticoids alone.[33] Alternative medications that can be used safely are acetaminophen at doses up to 650 mg, being aware that 20% of patients react to a dose of 1000 mg, or highly selective COX-2 inhibitors, such as celecoxib.[34] Aspirin desensitization in those instances where it is needed can be accomplished in nearly all patients with AERD, but once desensitized the patient must continue to take aspirin daily to maintain desensitized state.[35]

Nonselective β-blockers are another class of medication that present a problem to patients with asthma. In those with asthma, β-blockers cause increased bronchial obstruction and airway reactivity, and importantly blunt the effect of inhaled or oral β-receptor agonists, such as albuterol, which plays a key role in treatment of acute asthma exacerbations.[36] In most people with asthma without concomitant cardiovascular disease, routine use of even cardioselective β-blockers for treatment of hypertension is to be avoided.[37] Some studies have shown that in moderate and stable asthma, selective β-blockers may be used at low doses but require close physician supervision.[38] It is important for physicians to understand that although there is evidence to support using β-blockers to improve survival in patients with chronic obstructive pulmonary disease, possibly as a result of their cardiopulmonary protective properties, this does not currently apply to patients with asthma based on the most current review of the literature.[39]

Angiotensin-converting enzyme inhibitors deserve discussion because they relate to asthma triggers, primarily to point out that their most common side effect occurring at 5% to 20%, a dry hacking cough, can easily be mistaken for worsening asthma symptoms.[40] It is independent from asthma, and these patients should be switched to an angiotensin receptor blocker, which has a lower incidence of dry cough.

There are a plethora of inhaled irritants and pollutants that people with asthma should be made aware of that increase asthma exacerbations. These include, but are not limited to, tobacco smoke, fireplace smoke and ash, aerosols, perfumes, cooking odors, musty odors, shower steam, traffic pollution, air pollution, dust, and workplace irritants.[8]

Cigarette smoke is a well-studied airway irritant known to cause those with asthma to have more severe symptoms, increased rates of hospitalization, accelerated decline in lung function, and impaired response to inhaled and systemic glucocorticoids compared with nonsmokers.[41] Interestingly, in most developed countries approximately 25% of adults with asthma are current cigarette smokers, which is similar to the rate in the general population. This patient population presents unique issues in treatment in their reduced response to short-term corticosteroid therapy, which normally plays an important role in the typical treatment regimen. The mechanism of glucocorticoid resistance is not fully explained, but it has been postulated that it is caused by changes in airway inflammatory cell phenotypes, changes in glucocorticoid receptor alpha to beta ratio, and reduced histone deacetylase activity.[42] The strongest recommendation for smokers with asthma is to educate the patient about the various methods that are available to them to help them quit smoking as this best efficacy. It has been shown that by 6 weeks after smoking cessation considerable improvement in lung function and a fall in sputum neutrophil count occurs.[43] Unfortunately, it still remains difficult to maintain smoking cessation in people with asthma, as it is in all chronic smokers, and the only avenue is often trials of asthma drugs other than or in addition to glucocorticoids. There is some preliminary data that leukotriene-receptor antagonists may benefit smokers with mild asthma.[44]

PARADOXIC VOCAL FOLD DYSFUNCTION

Patients with this disorder can be acutely symptomatic and have even required intubation in the emergency setting. Once intubated, monitoring of their pulmonary functions demonstrates absolute normality. This is because the pathology of this asthma imposter is not the pulmonary tree but rather a paradoxic closure or adduction of the vocal cords on inspiration. Once intubated, the obstruction is bypassed. PVFD is usually present intermittently and may not be observed on video endoscopy of the larynx unless triggered by exercise or stress. A helpful diagnostic question is, "are you more short of breath on inspiration or expiration?". The patient with PVFD will answer "on breathing in," whereas the patient with asthma has problems with expiration. Breathing exercises and voice therapy can be helpful in treating PVFD.

EMOTIONAL TRIGGERS

Emotional states, such as stress and depression, are known to influence the level of asthma control.[8] Various studies have shown that children that grow up in more chronically stressful environments have higher prevalence of asthma.[45,46] A stronger correlation is seen between atopic asthma and stress, anxiety, and depression versus nonatopic asthma.[47] It is recommended that the emotional triggers in the patients be recognized and managed accordingly with the appropriate medications, psychotherapy, or social work to best alleviate the stressors.[8]

OBESITY

There is a positive correlation between obesity and increased prevalence and incidence of asthma and reduced asthma control.[1,48,49] A prospective cohort study of 86,000 individuals demonstrated a linear correlation between body mass index and adult-onset asthma incidence.[50] The mechanism is incompletely understood, but a significant portion is attributed to chronic low-grade systemic inflammation as a function of increased amounts of functioning adipose tissue resulting in release of various cytokines, chemokines, and the soluble fractions of their receptors. A recent study showed that there is increased eosinophilic activity associated with high serum leptin and tumor necrosis factor-α levels in atopic obese children and adolescents with asthma compared with nonobese healthy volunteers.[51] Mechanically, obese individuals have reduced lung function mechanics with decreased functional residual capacity, lung volume, and tidal volumes.[1] There are additionally the myriad comorbid conditions associated with obesity, such as dyslipidemia, GERD, type 2 diabetes, and hypertension, which further complicate management. It is recommended that all patients, not just those with asthma, be counseled about the benefits of weight loss and methods that are available to them.

RHINOSINUSITIS

In the last 15 years the unified airway model, with interrelatedness between the pathophysiologic processes of the upper airway and its influence on the lower airway, has shaped the therapy directed at both targets. It is known that nasal obstruction triggers asthma exacerbations and this is particularly problematic for those patients with nasal polyps. In pre-endoscopic and postendoscopic sinus surgery, review of 70 patients with chronic rhinosinusitis and concomitant asthma, improvement in symptoms and reduction in emergency room visits and medications resulted, whereas only two patients did not improve and required revision surgery for nasal polyps.[52]

In addition, the intense accumulation of inflammatory material in the sinuses is hypothesized to feed the fuel of lower airway inflammation, so improvement in chronic rhinosinusitis, either by establishing nasal breathing or by reducing inflammatory drip, can improve symptomatic asthma.

SUMMARY

The patient armed with knowledge about the disease process and how to identify triggers and exacerbating factors is best able to partner with the health care team to prevent exposure to triggers of asthmatic exacerbations and to control their symptoms. Important in treating and preventing asthma is the understanding that for many patients there is more than one trigger and there may be multiple triggers.

REFERENCES

1. National Asthma Education and Prevention Program. Expert panel report 3: guidelines for the diagnosis and management of asthma. Bethesda (MD): NIH publication: National Heart, Lung, and Blood Institute; 2007.
2. Ezratty V, Bonay M, Neukirch C, et al. Effect of formaldehyde on asthmatic response to inhaled allergen challenge. Environ Health Perspect 2007;115: 210–4.
3. Gannon PF, Bright P, Campbell M, et al. Occupational asthma due to glutaraldehyde and formaldehyde in endoscopy and X ray departments. Thorax 1995;50: 156–9.

4. Longo DL. 18th edition. Harrison's principles of internal medicine, vol. 2. New York: McGraw-Hill; 2012.

5. D'Amato G, Liccardi G, Frenguelli G. Thunderstorm-asthma and pollen allergy. Allergy 2007;62:11–6.

6. Siles RI, Hsieh FH. Allergy blood testing: a practical guide for clinicians. Cleve Clin J Med 2011;78:585–92.

7. Schwarze J, Gelfand EW. Respiratory viral infections as promoters of allergic sensitization and asthma in animal models. Eur Respir J 2002;19:341–9.

8. Bailey W, Miller R. Trigger control to enhance asthma management. In: Basow DS, editor. Waltham (MA): 2013.

9. Poole PJ, Chacko E, Wood-Baker RW, et al. Influenza vaccine for patients with chronic obstructive pulmonary disease. Cochrane Database Syst Rev 2006;(1):CD002733.

10. The safety of inactivated influenza vaccine in adults and children with asthma. N Engl J Med 2001;345:1529–36.

11. Harding SM. Recent clinical investigations examining the association of asthma and gastroesophageal reflux. Am J Med 2003;115(Suppl 3A):39S–44S.

12. Simpson WG. Gastroesophageal reflux disease and asthma. Diagnosis and Management. Arch Intern Med 1995;155:798–803.

13. Havemann BD, Henderson CA, El-Serag HB. The association between gastro-oesophageal reflux disease and asthma: a systematic review. Gut 2007;56: 1654–64.

14. Harding SM, Sontag SJ. Asthma and gastroesophageal reflux. Am J Gastroenterol 2000;95:S23–32.

15. Pearson JP, Parikh S, Orlando RC, et al. Review article: reflux and its consequences–the laryngeal, pulmonary and oesophageal manifestations. Conference held in conjunction with the 9th International Symposium on Human Pepsin (ISHP) Kingston-Upon-Hull, UK, 21-23 April 2010. Aliment Pharmacol Ther 2011;33(Suppl 1):1–71.

16. Schan CA, Harding SM, Haile JM, et al. Gastroesophageal reflux-induced bronchoconstriction. An intraesophageal acid infusion study using state-of-the-art technology. Chest 1994;106:731–7.

17. Vincent D, Cohen-Jonathan AM, Leport J, et al. Gastro-oesophageal reflux prevalence and relationship with bronchial reactivity in asthma. Eur Respir J 1997; 10:2255–9.

18. Littner MR, Leung FW, Ballard ED 2nd, et al, Lansoprazole Asthma Study Group. Effects of 24 weeks of lansoprazole therapy on asthma symptoms, exacerbations, quality of life, and pulmonary function in adult asthmatic patients with acid reflux symptoms. Chest 2005;128:1128–35.

19. Kiljander TO, Junghard O, Beckman O, et al. Effect of esomeprazole 40 Mg once or twice daily on asthma: a randomized, placebo-controlled study. Am J Respir Crit Care Med 2010;181:1042–8.

20. Centers American Lung Association Asthma Clinical Research, Mastronarde JG, Anthonisen NR, et al. Efficacy of esomeprazole for treatment of poorly controlled asthma. N Engl J Med 2009;360:1487–99.

21. Kiljander TO, Harding SM, Field SK, et al. Effects of esomeprazole 40 mg twice daily on asthma: a randomized placebo-controlled trial. Am J Respir Crit Care Med 2006;173:1091–7.

22. Kahrilas PJ, Shaheen NJ, Vaezi MF, American Gastroenterological Association Institute, Clinical Practice and Quality Management Committee. American Gastroenterological Association Institute technical review on the management

of gastroesophageal reflux disease. Gastroenterology 2008;135:1392–413, 1413.e1–5.

23. DeVault KR, Castell DO, American College of Gastroenterology. Updated guidelines for the diagnosis and treatment of gastroesophageal reflux disease. Am J Gastroenterol 2005;100:190–200.

24. Samter M, Beers RF Jr. Intolerance to aspirin. Clinical studies and consideration of its pathogenesis. Ann Intern Med 1968;68:975–83.

25. Hedman J, Kaprio J, Poussa T, et al. Prevalence of asthma, aspirin intolerance, nasal polyposis and chronic obstructive pulmonary disease in a population-based study. Int J Epidemiol 1999;28:717–22.

26. Jenkins C, Costello J, Hodge L. Systematic review of prevalence of aspirin induced asthma and its implications for clinical practice. BMJ 2004;328:434.

27. Weber RW, Hoffman M, Raine DA Jr, et al. Incidence of bronchoconstriction due to aspirin, azo dyes, non-azo dyes, and preservatives in a population of perennial asthmatics. J Allergy Clin Immunol 1979;64:32–7.

28. Dahlen B. Treatment of aspirin-intolerant asthma with antileukotrienes. Am J Respir Crit Care Med 2000;161:S137–41.

29. Israel E, Fischer AR, Rosenberg MA, et al. The pivotal role of 5-lipoxygenase products in the reaction of aspirin-sensitive asthmatics to aspirin. Am Rev Respir Dis 1993;148:1447–51.

30. Nasser SM, Bell GS, Foster S, et al. Effect of the 5-lipoxygenase inhibitor Zd2138 on aspirin-induced asthma. Thorax 1994;49:749–56.

31. Fahrenholz JM. Natural history and clinical features of aspirin-exacerbated respiratory disease. Clin Rev Allergy Immunol 2003;24:113–24.

32. Williams AN, Simon RA, Woessner KM, et al. The relationship between historical aspirin-induced asthma and severity of asthma induced during oral aspirin challenges. J Allergy Clin Immunol 2007;120:273–7.

33. Dahlen B, Nizankowska E, Szczeklik A, et al. Benefits from adding the 5-lipoxygenase inhibitor zileuton to conventional therapy in aspirin-intolerant asthmatics. Am J Respir Crit Care Med 1998;157:1187–94.

34. Settipane RA, Schrank PJ, Simon RA, et al. Prevalence of cross-sensitivity with acetaminophen in aspirin-sensitive asthmatic subjects. J Allergy Clin Immunol 1995;96:480–5.

35. Hope AP, Woessner KA, Simon RA, et al. Rational approach to aspirin dosing during oral challenges and desensitization of patients with aspirin-exacerbated respiratory disease. J Allergy Clin Immunol 2009;123:406–10.

36. Benson MK, Berrill WT, Cruickshank JM, et al. A comparison of four beta-adrenoceptor antagonists in patients with asthma. Br J Clin Pharmacol 1978;5:415–9.

37. Self TH, Wallace JL, Soberman JE. Cardioselective beta-blocker treatment of hypertension in patients with asthma: when do benefits outweigh risks? J Asthma 2012;49:947–51.

38. Sanfiorenzo C, Pipet A. Exacerbations of asthma–precipitating factors: drugs. Rev Mal Respir 2011;28:1059–70 [in French].

39. Rutten FH, Zuithoff NP, Hak E, et al. Beta-blockers may reduce mortality and risk of exacerbations in patients with chronic obstructive pulmonary disease. Arch Intern Med 2010;170:880–7.

40. Israili ZH, Hall WD. Cough and angioneurotic edema associated with angiotensin-converting enzyme inhibitor therapy. A review of the literature and pathophysiology. Ann Intern Med 1992;117:234–42.

41. Thomson NC, Chaudhuri R, Livingston E. Asthma and cigarette smoking. Eur Respir J 2004;24:822–33.

42. Thomson NC, Spears M. The influence of smoking on the treatment response in patients with asthma. Curr Opin Allergy Clin Immunol 2005;5:57–63.

43. Chaudhuri R, Livingston E, McMahon AD, et al. Effects of smoking cessation on lung function and airway inflammation in smokers with asthma. Am J Respir Crit Care Med 2006;174:127–33.

44. Thomson NC, Chaudhuri R. Asthma in smokers: challenges and opportunities. Curr Opin Pulm Med 2009;15:39–45.

45. Gupta RS, Zhang X, Springston EE, et al. The association between community crime and childhood asthma prevalence in Chicago. Ann Allergy Asthma Immunol 2010;104:299–306.

46. Pittman TP, Nykiforuk CI, Mignone J, et al. The association between community stressors and asthma prevalence of school children in Winnipeg, Canada. Int J Environ Res Public Health 2012;9:579–95.

47. Lind N, Nordin M, Palmquist E, et al. Psychological distress in asthma and allergy: the Vasterbotten Environmental Health Study. Psychol Health Med 2013. [Epub ahead of print].

48. Delgado J, Barranco P, Quirce S. Obesity and asthma. J Investig Allergol Clin Immunol 2008;18:420–5.

49. Taylor B, Mannino D, Brown C, et al. Body mass index and asthma severity in the national asthma survey. Thorax 2008;63:14–20.

50. Camargo CA Jr, Weiss ST, Zhang S, et al. Prospective study of body mass index, weight change, and risk of adult-onset asthma in women. Arch Intern Med 1999;159:2582–8.

51. Grotta MB, Squebola-Cola DM, Toro AA, et al. Obesity increases eosinophil activity in asthmatic children and adolescents. BMC Pulm Med 2013;13:39.

52. Nair S, Bhadauria RS, Sharma S. Effect of endoscopic sinus surgery on asthmatic patients with chronic rhinosinusitis. Indian J Otolaryngol Head Neck Surg 2010;62:285–8.

Exercise-induced Bronchoconstriction

Jonathan P. Parsons, MD, MSc

KEYWORDS

- Asthma • Exercise • Exercise-induced bronchoconstriction • Bronchoprovocation
- Diagnosis • Athletes • Treatment

KEY POINTS

- Exercise-induced bronchoconstriction (EIB) occurs in individuals with and without chronic asthma.
- The symptoms of EIB are often subtle and difficult to differentiate from normal manifestations of intense exercise.
- Diagnosis of EIB based on subjective symptoms alone is extremely inaccurate.
- Objective testing is strongly recommended to document a diagnosis of EIB.
- Treatment of EIB with a short-acting bronchodilator before exercise is 80% effective.
- If short-acting bronchodilators are used daily for prophylaxis, controller agents such as inhaled steroids should also be added.
- Adjunctive treatment approaches (adequate warm-up, allergen avoidance, dietary modification, etc.) may also be helpful.

INTRODUCTION

Exercise-induced bronchoconstriction (EIB) describes acute, transient airway narrowing that is provoked by exercise. EIB is characterized by symptoms of cough, wheezing, shortness of breath, fatigue, and/or chest tightness during or after exercise. Exercise is a very common trigger of bronchoconstriction in asthmatics, and 80% of all individuals with chronic asthma experience exercise-induced respiratory symptoms at some point.[1] EIB also occurs in up to 10% of subjects who are not known to be atopic or asthmatic.[2] This cohort does not have the typical features of chronic asthma (ie, nocturnal symptoms, multiple triggers, impaired lung function), and exercise may be the only trigger that causes such individuals respiratory symptoms.

EIB also occurs quite commonly in athletes, and prevalence rates of bronchoconstriction related to exercise in cohorts of athletes range from 11% to 50%.[3] This

Disclosures: Dr J.P. Parsons is a consultant for Teva, Inc.
Wexner Medical Center, The Ohio State University, 201 Davis Heart/Lung Research Institute, 473 West 12th Avenue, Columbus, OH 43210, USA
E-mail address: jonathan.parsons@osumc.edu

Otolaryngol Clin N Am 47 (2014) 119–126
http://dx.doi.org/10.1016/j.otc.2013.09.003   oto.theclinics.com

wide variability in reported prevalence rates, in part, is a consequence of variable testing methods, thresholds for diagnosis, and participant populations. EIB is prevalent in endurance sports in which ventilatory load is increased for extended periods of time during training and competition (ie, soccer, lacrosse, swimming, long-distance running)[4]; however, EIB can occur in any setting. EIB also occurs commonly in cold weather and winter sports athletes.[5] In addition, environmental triggers may predispose certain populations of athletes to an increased risk for development of EIB. Chloramine compounds in swimming pools[6] and chemicals related to ice-resurfacing machinery in ice rinks[7] may put exposed athletic populations at additional risk. Athletic fields in urban or high-traffic areas for vehicles may be more likely to cause EIB symptoms.[8]

Despite how prevalent EIB is, the actual prevalence of EIB may actually be underestimated for multiple reasons. Patients with asthma and EIB have been shown to be poor perceivers of symptoms of bronchospasm.[9,10] Athletes, specifically, often suffer from lack of awareness of symptoms suggestive of EIB.[11,12] Furthermore, if they do recognize they have a medical problem, they often do not want to admit to health personnel that a problem exists due to fear of social stigma or losing playing time.[13] In addition to this lack of self-perception, health care providers, parents, and coaches also may not consider EIB as a possible explanation for respiratory symptoms occurring during exercise. Athletes are generally fit and healthy and the presence of a significant medical problem often is not considered. The athlete is often considered to be "out of shape," and vague symptoms of chest discomfort, breathlessness, and fatigue are not interpreted as a pathologic problem.

DIAGNOSIS

The clinical manifestations of EIB are extremely variable and can range from impairment of athletic performance (most cases) to severe bronchospasm and respiratory failure (less common, yet still possible). Common symptoms include coughing, wheezing, chest tightness, and dyspnea. More subtle evidence of EIB includes fatigue, symptoms that occur in specific environments (eg, ice rinks or swimming pools), poor performance for conditioning level (running/swimming slower than expected times), and avoidance of activity (very common in school-aged children) (**Box 1**).

Generally, exercise at a workload representing at least 80% of the maximal predicted oxygen consumption for 5 to 8 minutes is required to generate an episode of EIB.[14] If the onset of symptoms occurs more quickly after starting exercise, then EIB is less likely. Typically, most people experience transient bronchodilation initially during exercise, and symptoms of EIB begin later or shortly after exercise. Symptoms may

---

Box 1
Common symptoms of EIB

Dyspnea on exertion

Chest tightness

Wheezing

Fatigue

Poor performance for conditioning level

Avoidance of activity

Symptoms in specific environments

manifest after exercise ceases and can remain significant for 30 minutes or longer if no bronchodilator therapy is provided.[15] Some patients spontaneously recover to baseline airflow within 60 minutes, even in the absence of intervention with bronchodilator therapy, which is clearly not recommended.[15] Individuals who experience symptoms for extended periods frequently perform at suboptimal levels for significant portions of their competitive or recreational activities.

The presence of EIB can be challenging to recognize clinically, because symptoms are often nonspecific. Complete history and physical examination should be performed on each patient with respiratory complaints associated with exercise. However, despite the value of a comprehensive history in the patient with exertional respiratory symptoms, the diagnosis of EIB based on self-reported symptoms alone has been shown to be extremely inaccurate[16]; this is likely due to the lack of specificity of symptoms and the fact that in most cases the physical examination will be normal. The poor predictive value of the history and physical examination in the evaluation of EIB strongly suggests that clinicians should perform objective diagnostic testing when there is a clinical suspicion of EIB.

Other medical problems that commonly mimic EIB and that need to be considered in the initial evaluation include vocal cord dysfunction, gastroesophageal reflux disease, and allergic rhinitis/sinus disease (**Box 2**). Cardiac pathology such as arrhythmia, cardiomyopathy, and cardiac shunts are much less common, but need to be considered as well. A comprehensive history and examination is recommended to help rule out these other disorders, and specific testing such as echocardiography, allergy testing, and/or videolaryngostroboscopy may be required. A history of specific symptoms in particular environments or during specific activities should be elicited. Timing of symptom onset in relation to exercise and recovery is also helpful.

Objective testing should begin with spirometry before and after inhaled bronchodilator therapy, which will help identify athletes whose lung function was impaired at rest. However, most people who experience EIB have normal baseline lung function.[17] In these patients, spirometry alone is not adequate to diagnose EIB. Significant numbers of false-negative results may occur if adequate exercise and environmental stress are not provided in the evaluation for EIB. In patients being evaluated for EIB who have a normal physical examination and normal spirometry, bronchoprovocation testing is recommended. A positive bronchoprovocation test indicates the need for treatment of EIB. A decrease of 10% or (greater forced expiratory volume in 1 second [FEV_1]) between pretest and post-test values is diagnostic of EIB.[16] In a patient with persistent exercise-related symptoms and negative physical examination, spirometry, and bronchoprovocation testing, alternative diagnoses other than EIB should be considered.

The International Olympic Committee recommends eucapnic voluntary hyperventilation (EVH) as the bronchoprovocation test of choice to document EIB in Olympians. EVH involves hyperventilation of a gas mixture of 5% CO_2 and 21% O_2 at a target

---

Box 2
Mimics of EIB

Vocal cord dysfunction

Gastroesophageal reflux disease

Allergic rhinitis/sinus disease

Cardiac pathology (arrhythmias, cardiomyopathy, shunts)

ventilation rate of 85% of the patient's maximal voluntary ventilation in 1 minute (MVV). The MVV is usually calculated as 35 times the baseline FEV_1. The patient continues to hyperventilate for 6 minutes, and assessment of FEV_1 occurs at specified intervals up to 20 minutes after the test. This challenge test has been shown to have a high specificity[18] for EIB. EVH has also been shown to be more sensitive for detecting EIB than methacholine[4] or field- or lab-based exercise testing.[18] However, the major limitation of EVH is that it is not widely available.

Mannitol inhalation is a newer bronchoprovocation technique that has been shown to be effective in diagnosing EIB in athletes. Mannitol inhalation is an osmotic airway challenge that involves inhaling mannitol at increasing concentrations (up to 160 mg). The test is terminated when the last dose of mannitol has been given or the FEV_1 has dropped 15% or greater from baseline. The mannitol challenge is portable and can be used for field, clinic, or laboratory testing to identify EIB. Mannitol inhalation correlates well with traditional exercise testing and EVH.[19] There are some potential limitations in using mannitol to identify airway hyperresponsiveness. As with any osmotic challenge, mannitol inhalation will frequently provoke a person to cough. Excessive coughing has the potential to affect the mannitol dose deposited in the lower airway, which could lead to a false-negative test result.[20]

Treadmill or ergometer-based testing in pulmonary function laboratories are effective methods for diagnosing EIB but may result in false-negatives if the exercise stimulus is not intense enough. The optimal exercise challenge is 8 minutes in duration and allows the patient to achieve greater than 90% of maximum predicted heart rate by 2 minutes into the challenge and maintain it for the remaining 6 minutes of the challenge.[21,22]

Field-exercise challenge tests that involve athletes performing the sport in which they are normally involved and assessing lung function pre- and post-exercise have been shown to be less sensitive than EVH[23] and allow for little standardization of a protocol.

Pharmacologic challenge tests, such as the methacholine challenge test, have been shown to have a lower sensitivity than EVH for detection of EIB in athletes[16] and are also not recommended for first-line evaluation of EIB (**Table 1**).

Table 1
Comparison of testing modalities for EIB

Test	Comments
Eucapnic voluntary hyperventilation	• Generally accepted as the recommended test to document EIB • Not widely available
Laboratory-based exercise testing	• Most common test used to document EIB • Widely available • Must ensure the exercise stimulus is intense enough to avoid false–negative results
Field-based exercise testing	• Low sensitivity to diagnose EIB • Usually informal and does not utilize protocols
Mannitol inhalation	• Portable • Commonly induces cough, which may lead to inadequate/false-negative tests • Not widely available
Methacholine challenge	• Very poor specificity for EIB • Not recommended for evaluation of EIB

PHARMACOLOGIC THERAPY

The most common therapeutic recommendation to minimize or prevent symptoms of EIB is the prophylactic use of a short-acting β-agonist (SABA) such as albuterol shortly before exercise.[24] Treatment with 2 puffs of a SABA before exercise (15–20 minutes) will provide peak bronchodilation in 15 to 60 minutes and protection from EIB for at least 3 hours in most patients. Over time, frequent use of prophylactic SABA may lead to tachyphylaxis. As a result, an additional controller agent such as inhaled corticosteroid is generally added whenever prophylactic SABA therapy is used daily or more frequently.[16]

Long-acting bronchodilators work in a similar manner pharmacologically as short-acting bronchodilators; however, the bronchoprotection afforded by long-acting β-agonists has been shown to last up to 12 hours. However, tachyphylaxis also has been shown to occur after repeated use of long-acting β-agonists.[25] In addition, recent guidelines recommend against daily use of an inhaled long-acting β-agonist as *single* therapy based on a strong concern for serious side effects.[16]

Inhaled corticosteroids (ICS) are first-line therapy in terms of controller medications for patients who have chronic asthma and also experience EIB.[24] ICS are taken daily and are not used in a prophylactic manner before exercise. It may take 2 to 4 weeks after the initiation of therapy to see maximal improvement.

Leukotriene modifiers have also been shown to be effective in treating EIB.[26] Leukotriene modifiers, such as montelukast, given once daily, will reduce EIB and also improve the recovery to baseline. There is no development of tolerance when taken daily.[27] If montelukast is used prophylactically for EIB, it needs to be taken 2 hours before planned exercise.

Mast cell stabilizers or cromolyn compounds have been studied extensively for the prophylaxis of EIB. These medications prevent mast cell degranulation and subsequent histamine release. Although these agents are effective, they are often used as a second-line treatment because of their cost, lack of availability in the United States, and their decreased duration of action and efficacy compared with SABA.

NONPHARMACOLOGIC THERAPY

Many individuals find that a period of preexercise warm-up reduces the risk of EIB occurring during their subsequent exercise session. It has been shown by investigators that this refractory period does occur in some people and that they can be refractory to an exercise task performed within 2 hours of an exercise warm-up.[28,29] However, the refractory period has not been consistently proved across different athletic populations, and it is currently not possible to identify who will experience this refractory period.[30]

Other nonpharmacologic strategies can be used to help reduce the frequency and severity of symptoms of EIB. Breathing through the nose rather than the mouth will also help attenuate EIB[31] by warming, filtering, and humidifying the air, which subsequently reduces airway cooling and dehydration. Wearing a face-mask/scarf during activity warms and humidifies inspired air when outdoor conditions are cold and dry and is especially valuable to elite and recreational athletes who exercise in the winter.[32] In addition, people with knowledge of triggers (eg, freshly cut grass) should attempt to avoid them if possible. Dietary modifications including low-salt diet, or ascorbic acid and/or fish-oil supplementation may reduce the risk or severity of EIB.[33–35] These studies are small and need to be confirmed in larger trials, but may be effective adjunctive management strategies with negligible associated risk (**Table 2**).

Table 2
Treatment of EIB

Pharmacologic Therapy	Nonpharmacologic Therapy
Short-acting β-agonists • 1st-line prophylactic therapy	Adequate preexercise warm-up
Inhaled corticosteroids • 1st-line controller therapy	Wearing a mask/scarf in cold environment
Long-acting β-agonists • Not recommended as monotherapy	Avoidance of triggers
Leukotriene modifiers • If used prophylactically, must be dosed 2 h before exercise	Nasal breathing
Cromolyn compounds • Not widely available in the United States	Dietary modification (low-salt, Vitamin C, fish oil)

SUMMARY

EIB is prevalent, particularly in people with asthma and in populations of athletes. The diagnosis of EIB based on symptoms alone is extremely inaccurate. Objective testing is necessary to make a confident diagnosis of EIB. EVH is considered by many to be the bronchoprovocation test of choice to document EIB; however, EVH may not be available to many health care providers. If EVH is not easily accessible, spirometry before and after an adequate exercise challenge is the next best option. It is essential to ensure that the exercise challenge is strenuous enough to generate adequate ventilation rates in patients who have excellent physical fitness.

Both pharmacologic and nonpharmacologic approaches are essential to minimize the adverse effects of EIB. Athletes who have clinical evidence of EIB should be treated with short-acting bronchodilators before exercise. This regimen will prevent significant EIB in more than 80% of athletes. If athletes use SABA daily for prophylaxis, it is recommended that a controller agent such as inhaled corticosteroid be added in addition. If symptoms persist, especially in athletes with asthma, the authors recommend adding inhaled corticosteroids as maintenance therapy. Alternatively, leukotriene modifiers or cromolyn compounds can be used in athletes inadequately controlled with β_2-agonists.

REFERENCES

1. Parsons JP, Craig TJ, Stoloff SW, et al. Impact of exercise-related respiratory symptoms in adults with asthma: Exercise-Induced Bronchospasm Landmark National Survey. Allergy Asthma Proc 2011;32(6):431–7.
2. Gotshall RW. Exercise-induced bronchoconstriction. Drugs 2002;62(12):1725–39.
3. Rundell KW, Jenkinson DM. Exercise-induced bronchospasm in the elite athlete. Sports Med 2002;32(9):583–600.
4. Holzer K, Anderson SD, Douglass J. Exercise in elite summer athletes: challenges for diagnosis. J Allergy Clin Immunol 2002;110(3):374–80.
5. Wilber RL, et al. Incidence of exercise-induced bronchospasm in Olympic winter sport athletes. Med Sci Sports Exerc 2000;32(4):732–7.
6. Helenius IJ, Rytila P, Metso T, et al. Respiratory symptoms, bronchial responsiveness, and cellular characteristics of induced sputum in elite swimmers. Allergy 1998;53(4):346–52.

7. Rundell KW. High levels of airborne ultrafine and fine particulate matter in indoor ice arenas. Inhal Toxicol 2003;15(3):237–50.
8. Rundell KW, Caviston R, Hollenbach AM, et al. Vehicular air pollution, playgrounds, and youth athletic fields. Inhal Toxicol 2006;18(8):541–7.
9. Barnes PJ. Poorly perceived asthma. Thorax 1992;47(6):408–9.
10. Barnes PJ. Blunted perception and death from asthma. N Engl J Med 1994; 330(19):1383–4.
11. Rundell KW, Im J, Mayers LB, et al. Self-reported symptoms and exercise-induced asthma in the elite athlete. Med Sci Sports Exerc 2001;33(2): 208–13.
12. Thole RT, Sallis RE, Rubin AL, et al. Exercise-induced bronchospasm prevalence in collegiate cross-country runners. Med Sci Sports Exerc 2001;33(10): 1641–6.
13. Moran W. Jackie Joyner-Kersee races against asthma. USA Today 2002.
14. Parsons JP, Mastronarde JG. Exercise-induced bronchoconstriction in athletes. Chest 2005;128(6):3966–74.
15. Brudno DS, Wagner JM, Rupp NT. Length of postexercise assessment in the determination of exercise-induced bronchospasm. Ann Allergy 1994;73(3):227–31.
16. Parsons JP, Hallstrand TS, Mastronarde JG, et al. An official American thoracic society clinical practice guideline: exercise-induced bronchoconstriction. Am J Respir Crit Care Med 2013;187(9):1016–27.
17. Rundell KW, Wilber RL, Szmedra L, et al. Exercise-induced asthma screening of elite athletes: field versus laboratory exercise challenge. Med Sci Sports Exerc 2000;32(2):309–16.
18. Eliasson AH, Phillips YY, Rajagopal KR, et al. Sensitivity and specificity of bronchial provocation testing. An evaluation of four techniques in exercise-induced bronchospasm. Chest 1992;102(2):347–55.
19. Cockcroft D, Davis B. Direct and indirect challenges in the clinical assessment of asthma. Ann Allergy Asthma Immunol 2009;103(5):363–9 [quiz: 369–72, 400].
20. Brannan JD, Anderson SD, Perry CP, et al. The safety and efficacy of inhaled dry powder mannitol as a bronchial provocation test for airway hyperresponsiveness: a phase 3 comparison study with hypertonic (4.5%) saline. Respir Res 2005;6:144.
21. Anderson SD, Argyros GJ, Magnussen H, et al. Provocation by eucapnic voluntary hyperpnoea to identify exercise induced bronchoconstriction. Br J Sports Med 2001;35(5):344–7.
22. Rundell KW, Slee JB. Exercise and other indirect challenges to demonstrate asthma or exercise-induced bronchoconstriction in athletes. J Allergy Clin Immunol 2008; 122(2):238–46 [quiz: 247–8].
23. Mannix ET, Manfredi F, Farber MO. A comparison of two challenge tests for identifying exercise-induced bronchospasm in figure skaters. Chest 1999;115(3): 649–53.
24. National Asthma Education and Prevention Program. Expert Panel Report 3 (EPR-3): Guidelines for the Diagnosis and Management of Asthma-Summary Report 2007. J Allergy Clin Immunol 2007;120(Suppl 5):S94–138.
25. Ferrari M, Segattini C, Zanon R, et al. Comparison of the protective effect of formoterol and of salmeterol against exercise-induced bronchospasm when given immediately before a cycloergometric test. Respiration 2002;69(6):509–12.
26. Philip G, Villaran C, Pearlman DS, et al. Protection against exercise-induced bronchoconstriction two hours after a single oral dose of montelukast. J Asthma 2007; 44(3):213–7.

27. Edelman JM, Turpin JA, Bronsky EA, et al. Oral montelukast compared with inhaled salmeterol to prevent exercise-induced bronchoconstriction. A randomized, double-blind trial. Exercise Study Group. Ann Intern Med 2000;132(2): 97–104.

28. Anderson SD, Schoeffel RE. Respiratory heat and water loss during exercise in patients with asthma. Effect of repeated exercise challenge. Eur J Respir Dis 1982;63(5):472–80.

29. McKenzie DC, McLuckie SL, Stirling DR. The protective effects of continuous and interval exercise in athletes with exercise-induced asthma. Med Sci Sports Exerc 1994;26(8):951–6.

30. Rundell KW, Spiering BA, Judelson DA, et al. Bronchoconstriction during cross-country skiing: is there really a refractory period? Med Sci Sports Exerc 2003; 35(1):18–26.

31. Shturman-Ellstein R, Zeballos RJ, Buckley JM, et al. The beneficial effect of nasal breathing on exercise-induced bronchoconstriction. Am Rev Respir Dis 1978; 118(1):65–73.

32. Schachter EN, Lach E, Lee M. The protective effect of a cold weather mask on exercised-induced asthma. Ann Allergy 1981;46(1):12–6.

33. Mickleborough TD, Gotshall RW. Dietary salt intake as a potential modifier of airway responsiveness in bronchial asthma. J Altern Complement Med 2004; 10(4):633–42.

34. Mickleborough TD, Ionescu AA, Rundell KW. Omega-3 Fatty acids and airway hyperresponsiveness in asthma. J Altern Complement Med 2004;10(6):1067–75.

35. Tecklenburg SL, Mickleborough TD, Fly AD, et al. Ascorbic acid supplementation attenuates exercise-induced bronchoconstriction in patients with asthma. Respir Med 2007;101(8):1770–8.

Patient Education and Designing an Asthma Action Plan

Elizabeth Boise, RNC, BSN, AE-C

KEYWORDS

- Asthma • Patient education • Asthma assessment • Asthma action plan
- Asthma symptom management • Teaching moment • Asthma control

KEY POINTS

- It is essential to ask precise questions to elicit the most accurate clinical information from patients.
- Written asthma symptom and medication usage tracking sheets should be used to monitor compliance and asthma control.
- Quality of care for asthma and allergy patients may be improved through consistent asthma "detective" work.
- Asthma/allergy patients should be coached toward better control and an improved quality of life.
- Patients' risk of anaphylaxis is decreased by providing an in-depth asthma assessment before allergy skin testing.

INTRODUCTION

In the Oto-Allergy Clinic at the Ohio State University Wexner Medical Center, Department of Otolaryngology, Division of Sinus and Allergy, we strive to provide the best asthma care we can within the constraints of our practice. By networking with others, learning what other offices have tried and what works, attending the American Academy of Otolaryngic Allergy training courses, and reviewing the 2007 National Institutes of Health (NIH) guidelines for the diagnosis and treatment of asthma, we gather valuable information to improve our standard of care for our allergy and asthma patients. Applying these best practice principles takes additional time and staff training. Quality, coordinated, and effective asthma care can be accomplished in every office with a few small changes to the way you assess your patients. We have had many patients ask us

The author has no disclosures.
Division of Sinus and Allergy, OSU Department of Otolaryngology – Head and Neck Surgery, Wexner Medical Center at The Ohio State University, 915 Olentangy River Road, Suite 4000, Columbus, OH 43212, USA
E-mail address: elizabeth.boise@osumc.edu

Otolaryngol Clin N Am 47 (2014) 127–134
http://dx.doi.org/10.1016/j.otc.2013.09.008

Abbreviations	
ACT	Asthma control test
AAP	Asthma action plan
FENO	Fractional exhaled nitric oxide
HEPA	High-efficiency particulate air
NHLBI	National Heart, Lung, and Blood Institute
NIH	National Institutes of Health
PEF	Peak expiratory flow

why we are asking so many questions and doing several breathing tests when "no one else has done them."

Our patients who seek our care deserve the best possible: to breathe well and to be able to do what everyone else can do who does not have asthma. We love hearing: "I didn't really know what feeling good was until I came here." Improving a patient's quality of life makes the extra effort very worthwhile.

The NIH Guidelines on Asthma were developed by an expert panel commissioned by the National Asthma Education and Prevention Program Coordinating Committee, coordinated by the National Heart, Lung, and Blood Institute (NHLBI) of the National Institutes of Health to improve the quality of an asthma patient's care. The expert panel identified 4 essential components of asthma care:

- Assessment and monitoring
- Patient education
- Control of factors contributing to asthma severity
- Pharmacologic treatment

One of the NIH guideline's goals in asthma therapy is to achieve asthma control by reducing the patient's impairment and risk, providing periodic clinical and self-assessments, using minimally invasive markers such as spirometry, and providing a written asthma action plan (AAP) based on signs and symptoms or peak expiratory flow (PEF) readings.

We would like to share how we try to incorporate these guidelines into our everyday practice provide in-depth and ongoing patient education, as well as how to develop coordinated plans to improve our patient's health.

THE OTO-ALLERGY CLINIC ASTHMA ASSESSMENT

In our Oto-Allergy Clinic, we actively look for undiagnosed and uncontrolled asthma in each of our patients. Many come to us seeking help for their "allergies," when their underlying problem is actually undiagnosed asthma. This type of "detective" work is time consuming, but the rewards great when you see your patient's quality of life improve.

We believe the extra effort is worthwhile because asthma still affects more than 25 million Americans, causes almost 3400 deaths per year, and costs more than $56 billion in annual health care costs. We screen all patients carefully, because someone with uncontrolled or undiagnosed asthma has a higher incidence of having anaphylaxis, a severe allergic reaction, when we perform allergy testing.

ASKING THE RIGHT QUESTIONS

When assessing our patients at their initial visit, we ask if they have a history of asthma and/or have had a cough, chest tightness, wheezing, or shortness of breath. If they answer yes, can they pinpoint what exposure caused their symptoms? Was it a certain time of year (spring, fall, or year-round)? Was it when they came in contact with a certain substance or animal?

With pet allergies, patients can usually easily relate their symptoms to when they touched a certain animal or were in a house with that animal. Approximately half of asthma is allergic asthma, so determining their allergic asthma triggers is paramount in exposure prevention and sequential allergy treatment.

THE ASTHMA CONTROL TEST

If the patient states that they have a history of asthma, we encourage them to complete an Asthma Control Test (ACT). There are many versions of this short questionnaire available that you can use. It aims at identifying how asthma is affecting their everyday life. Patients fill out the ACT while waiting for their physician. It only takes a few minutes and gives us valuable information about a patient's asthma control.

The ACT asks: How often in the past 4 weeks
- Have you had recurrent coughing, shortness of breath, wheezing, or chest tightness?
- Have you used your rescue inhaler or nebulizer (Albuterol)?
- Have you been awakened at night by asthma symptoms?
- Has your asthma kept you from getting as much done as usual at school, work, or home?
- Have you been to the Emergency Department because of your asthma?

The ACT is a reliable, valid tool to help physicians identify patients with uncontrolled asthma and to help follow a patient's progress with their treatment. Returning patients with asthma complete the ACT at each subsequent visit. The physician then reviews these results before seeing the patient. Another quick way you can assess a patient's asthma control is with the "Rules of Two."

- In the last week have you used your rescue inhaler more than 2 times?
- In the last month have you been awakened by your asthma more than 2 times?
- Have you refilled your rescue inhalers more than 2 times in the last year?

It is important to determine the frequency of the patient's symptoms and relate these symptoms to what was happening to the patient at the time. We must ask the right questions to get an accurate assessment of the frequency and severity of symptoms that they have been experiencing.

If you ask your patient how their asthma is, they will often answer, "Fine." If you ask how many times in the last week/month they have used their rescue inhaler, you will get another answer. More precisely, if you ask how many times your patient has had cough, chest tightness, wheezing, or shortness of breath, you will get even more information. Asking the right questions is one of the most important things we can do to gather all the "clues" we need to solve the mystery of why they are feeling the way they do.

Patients often have asthma symptoms but will not use their rescue inhaler, even though they should. Oftentimes they have lived with these symptoms for so long and do not recognize them as abnormal. If they do not have an accurate perception of their airflow, it is a risk factor for death from asthma. We have had patients say that the inhaler did not help or that they did not have one when their symptoms occurred. This situation is an important teaching moment, where you can verify if they primed their inhaler (must be primed if not used in 14 days), if they were using the rescue inhaler or their controller medication, or if they used enough medication

(2 puffs) as directed. Asthma assessment should be done with every patient interaction.

Sometimes, patients are given a prescription for an inhaler and never taught how to use their device. It only takes a minute to demonstrate proper inhaler technique and, if a patient was given a sample, have them practice using it before going home. Sending them home with written instructions will also reinforce your teaching. The companies that make the asthma medications will give your office demonstration devices for you to teach patients on the proper technique to use their medication correctly.

For patients with asthma, we ask specifically how often they are taking their controller medication (if they are on one). We have them bring out their medications to verify which one they think to be their controller, as we have occasionally found that the patient is unsure. Providing printed clear labels with the words: *Controller and Rescue* and placing them on their medication devices helps clarify which one is which.

USING FRACTIONAL EXHALED NITRIC OXIDE

At our institution all patients complete a fractional exhaled nitric oxide (FENO) measurement to

- Diagnose airway inflammation (eosinophilic)
- Determine the likelihood of corticosteroid responsiveness in patients with chronic respiratory symptoms possibly due to airway inflammation
- Support the diagnosis of asthma
- Monitor airway inflammation in patients who have asthma

This is a small hand-held domed device that the patient inhales and then exhales into through a special filtered mouthpiece to obtain a reading. The results are obtained in less than 1.5 minutes. We like to see a normal reading of less than 25. Results higher than 25 may require treatment and follow-up care.

The reason this measurement is important is that nitric oxide is a marker of airway inflammation. FENO provides information on which patients have allergic inflammation, whether a patient is taking their inhaled corticosteroid, if their prescribed therapy is working and if there has been a change in their allergen exposure.

If the patient's results are elevated, we use this teaching moment to review their medication compliance and allergen exposure.

PEAK EXPIRATORY FLOW

Next, patients have their PEF measured. PEF is a screening measure of the airflow through the bronchial tubes and helps determine if there is obstruction in the airways.

Our hand-held peak flow meter uses low-cost filtered disposable mouthpieces and is simple to use. PEF is very effort dependent so the patient needs adequate coaching to get an accurate measurement. It is recommended to keep a tape measure in the examination room to obtain an accurate height of the patient. The normal range is determined by the patient's age, height, and gender. This range is used to complete their AAP later.

SPIROMETRY

If the patient's PEF reading is below average, and the patient has a history of asthma or has any asthma symptoms, then we perform spirometry (pre- and post-bronchodilator). We use Albuterol via nebulizer or 4 puffs via a metered dose inhaler with a disposable mouthpiece. Trained coaching is needed to achieve accurate spirometry measurements. It is not difficult to learn; it just takes practice. The 2007 NIH guidelines recommend spirometry to be completed on all asthma patients at the time of their initial visit, after treatment has begun and symptoms and PEF have normalized, and during exacerbations. Follow-up spirometry should be done every 1 to 2 years.

We have large asthma posters on the examination room walls and encourage patients to read them while waiting or doing a nebulizer treatment. Asthma information on posters is an efficient way to incorporate asthma education into their visit. Later, the spirometry results are reviewed with the patient, who is given a copy of their own to take home (**Box 1**).

The peak flow reading, FENO measurement, spirometry, patient symptom history, and physical examination are all used to identify and diagnose our patients with asthma. Because patients with undiagnosed or uncontrolled asthma have an increased risk of anaphylaxis with allergy skin-prick and intradermal testing, it is imperative all patients are screened thoroughly before testing. If the patient is diagnosed with asthma, they are often sent home with an inhaled corticosteroid for 4 to 6 weeks, a rescue inhaler, and are scheduled to return for a follow-up. Allergy skin testing is deferred until their asthma is controlled.

It is a good practice to customize and send patients home with a written AAP (**Fig. 1**). There are several versions of the AAP available from the American Lung Association, the NHLBI, and respiratory companies, or you can create your own. It helps patients to have written instructions at home of how to self-manage their asthma and when to call their doctor. We have a copy of the AAP scanned into our electronic medical record.

ASTHMA TRIGGER AVOIDANCE EDUCATION

Because allergies are a common asthma trigger, we must educate our patients how to identify and avoid these triggers. Asthma trigger avoidance education includes:

- Dust mites: Use special allergen covers on mattresses and pillows. Wash pillows, stuffed animals, and linens in 130° to 140° water weekly. Treat or remove bedroom carpets and treat furniture for dust mites. Use high-efficiency particulate air (HEPA) filtration, especially in the bedroom. Use a HEPA vacuum.
- Animal dander: We do not tell patients that they have to get rid of their pets, but instead advise patients to bathe their pets at least weekly, use HEPA air filtration (especially in the bedroom), and keep the pet out of the bedroom. If the pet is a trigger, it is advised to avoid the pet as much as possible and to use a HEPA

Box 1
Contraindications to spirometry

- Recent thoracic or abdominal surgery
- Thoracic, cerebral, or abdominal aneurysm
- Unstable cardiovascular status
- Pneumothorax
- Hemoptysis
- Recent eye surgery
- Presence of acute disease

Asthma Action Plan

For: _____ Date: _____ Doctor: Karen Calhoun 614-366-3687, For Emergency call: **911**

Green Zone: Doing Well
- No cough, wheeze, chest tightness, or shortness of breath during the day or night
- Can do usual activities
- Peak flow: more than _____ (80 % or more of my best peak flow). My best peak flow is: _____

Take these long-term control medicines each day:

Medicine	How much to take	When to take it
		Daily

Take Albuterol (Rescue) Inhaler, 2 puffs, 10 to 20 minutes before exercise if you have exercise-induced asthma.

Yellow Zone: Asthma Is Getting Worse

- Cough, wheeze, chest tightness, or shortness of breath, or
- Waking at night due to asthma, or
- Can do some, but not all, usual activities, or
- Peak flow: _____ to _____(50 to 79 % of my best peak flow)

First: Take your quick-relief medicine: **Albuterol Inhaler 2 to 4 puffs** now (Keep taking your GREEN ZONE medicine)
Second: If your symptoms (and peak flow) return to your GREEN ZONE after 1 hour of above treatment:
   Continue monitoring to be sure you stay in the green zone.
If your symptoms (and peak flow) do not return to your GREEN ZONE after 1 hour of above treatment:
Take: Your short-acting beta$_2$-agonist: **Albuterol 2 to 4 puffs every 20 minutes for up to 1 hour**
       Your oral steroid: **Prednisone 10 mg, by mouth**, once per day for ____ days, if prescribed
       Call your doctor.

Red Zone: Medical Alert!
- Very short of breath, trouble walking and talking due to shortness of breath or
- Quick-relief medicines have not helped, or
- Cannot do usual activities, or
- Lips or fingernails are blue, or
- Symptoms are same or get worse after 24 hours in Yellow Zone, or
- Peak flow: is less than _____ (50 % of my best peak flow)

Take: Your Quick-relief medicine: **Albuterol inhaler 4 to 6 puffs**
       Your oral steroid: **Prednisone 10 mg, by mouth**, once, if prescribed
Go to the hospital or call an ambulance (911) if: You are still in your red zone after 15 minutes

*Example is from the NHLBI

Fig. 1. Example of an AAP from the NHLBI. (*Adapted from* National Heart, Lung, and Blood Institute. Asthma Action Plan. Available at: http://www.nhlbi.nih.gov/health/public/lung/asthma/asthma_actplan.pdf. Accessed September 9, 2013.)

vacuum. If a patient cannot control his or her asthma because of the pet, it is recommended that the patient finds a new home for the animal.
- Cockroach allergen: Use roach traps or sprays. Do not leave food out and keep your home clean.
- Tobacco smoke: Do not smoke and avoid being around smoke. Campfires and wood-burning stoves can irritate also.
- Pollens: Use HEPA air filtration, especially in the bedroom. Use saline sinus rinse, change clothes, and shower after exposure. Use air conditioning if possible. Stay indoors and keep windows closed when the pollen count is high (mid day and afternoon).
- Molds: Use HEPA air filtration, especially in the bedroom. Keep humidity less than 50%. Use dehumidifiers in damp areas. Keep bathrooms, kitchens, and basements well aired and clean. Clean up visible mold.
- Colds and infections: Avoid people with colds or the flu. Wash your hands frequently. Have a yearly flu shot.
- Medications: Some patients with asthma are sensitive to aspirin and other anti-inflammatory drugs. Avoid medications such as beta-blockers. Check with your physician or pharmacist on your medications.
- Exercise: Premedicate with your rescue inhaler 20 minutes before exercising. Warm up and cool down slowly.
- Weather: Wrap a scarf around your face when outside on cold or windy days.

- Strong emotions: Clearing your head and breathing deeply; see their primary care doctor for further management if needed.
- Strong odors, perfume: Avoid.

By asking our patients what causes their asthma symptoms and reviewing their asthma tracking sheets on their return visits, we can help them identify what their asthma triggers are and teach them how to avoid them. Because allergies are a common asthma trigger, we reinforce diligent allergy avoidance and use of their allergy medication as prescribed until their breathing is good enough to do allergy skin testing to determine what exact allergies they have. Using these avoidance techniques can help their asthma symptoms also.

PATIENT EDUCATION FOLDERS

Patients are sent home with bi-fold folders with pertinent asthma and allergy information. One side focuses on asthma; the other side focuses on allergy avoidance and may include:

• Understanding the respiratory system	• Asthma action plan
• Asthma trigger control plan	• Creating an allergy- free bedroom
• What is asthma?	• Dust mite allergy
• Asthma medications	• HEPA air filtration
• How to use your inhalers	• Mold allergy
• Over-the-counter antihistamines and eye drops	• Asthma symptom and medication tracking sheets

CUSTOMIZED ASTHMA SYMPTOM AND MEDICATION USE TRACKING SHEETS

Patients are sent home with our tracking sheets to self-monitor PEF, asthma symptoms, and medication compliance until their next visit (**Fig. 2**). These tracking sheets help us to identify a patient's asthma control quickly and increase the amount of specific information we obtain.

When patients return for their next visit, we repeat PEF, FENO, ACT, and/or spirometry as needed, review their asthma symptom tracking sheets, continue asthma education, and assess their asthma control. When their asthma is stabilized, we perform allergy skin testing to identify their allergic triggers. After identifying the causes of their symptoms, education is provided in avoidance of these triggers, how to use allergy symptom relief medications, and the availability of immunotherapy in the form of allergy drops or shots to make a permanent change in their immune system.

Ongoing documentation of your teaching and the patient's learning is helpful for continuity of care. Electronic medical records often do not have the templates that we need to document our teaching. Working with your computer department to develop these documents in ongoing flow sheets saves the staff time and allows quick access to the patient's progress. Until then, a copy of their education and tracking sheets can be scanned into the electronic medical records for further review.

Enlisting the patient's buy-in for self-monitoring and control will help them become an active member in their asthma care and improve compliance. Scheduling a patient for an asthma education visit (if you have an asthma educator in your office) can facilitate assessment of their understanding of their disease and where we need to concentrate further in their treatment plan. Also, by having a member of your staff

Week 1	Sun		Mon		Tues		Wed		Thurs		Fri		Sat	
	AM	PM	AM	PM	AM	PM	AM	PM	AM	PM	AM	PM	AM	PM
PEF														
Having cough, chest tightness, wheezing or shortness of breath? (C,CT,W, SOB)														
What was going on?														
Used rescue inhaler, 2 puffs? Helped?														
Controller medication taken daily?														
Triggers:														

Fig. 2. Tracking sheet for self-monitoring PEF, asthma symptoms, and medication compliance until next visit.

go through the additional training needed to be a certified asthma educator demonstrates your commitment to improving the quality of asthma care in your office.

FURTHER READINGS

American Lung Association. Available at: www.lung.org. Accessed October 23, 2013.
An Official ATS Clinical Practice Guideline: Interpretation of Exhaled Nitric Oxide Levels (FENO) for Clinical Applications.
National Asthma Education and Prevention Program Expert Panel Report 3. Guidelines for the Diagnosis and Management of Asthma 2007. NIH Publication Number 08-5846.

Paradoxic Vocal Fold Movement Disorder

Laura Matrka, MD[a,b,*]

KEYWORDS

- Vocal cord dysfunction • Paradoxical vocal fold movement disorder
- Paradoxical vocal cord movement disorder • Paradoxical vocal fold dysfunction
- Paradoxical vocal cord dysfunction • Paradoxical vocal fold motion dysfunction
- Paradoxical vocal cord motion dysfunction • Respiratory retraining therapy

KEY POINTS

- Paradoxic vocal fold movement disorder is more common than previously recognized and should be considered when dyspnea is present without pulmonary disease or out of proportion to the degree of coexistent pulmonary disease.
- Laryngeal control therapy (also called respiratory retraining therapy) with a speech language pathologist is the cornerstone of treatment of paradoxic vocal fold movement disorder.
- Flexible laryngoscopy must be performed to diagnose paradoxic vocal fold movement disorder. Laryngeal control therapy techniques should be trialed during this initial scope.
- Bilateral vocal fold paralysis, subglottic stenosis and tracheal stenosis must be ruled out, particularly when stridor is present.
- Comorbidities, such as laryngopharyngeal reflux, sinus or allergy problems, laryngeal sicca, and obstructive sleep apnea, should be identified and treated.
- Attention to controlling anxiety and stress levels is important. However, the role for counseling or psychiatric care in treating paradoxic vocal fold movement disorder may be decreasing as the contribution of medical comorbidities becomes more widely recognized.

INTRODUCTION

The first hint of paradoxic vocal fold movement disorder (PVFMD) in the medical literature came in 1842, in which a patient with "hysteric croup" was described.[1] The paradoxic movement itself was first visualized via laryngoscopy in 1869 by Mackenzie,[2] who

I have no financial disclosures to report.

[a] Department of Otolaryngology – Head and Neck Surgery, The Ohio State University Wexner Medical Center, Eye and Ear Institue, Suite 4000, 915 Olentangy River Road, Columbus, OH 43212, USA; [b] JamesCare Voice and Swallowing Disorders Clinic, Stoneridge Medical Center, 4019 West Dublin-Granville Road, Dublin, OH 43017, USA

* Department of Otolaryngology – Head and Neck Surgery, The Ohio State University Wexner Medical Center, Eye and Ear Institue, Suite 4000, 915 Olentangy River Road, Columbus, OH 43212.

E-mail address: Laura.matrka@osumc.edu

Otolaryngol Clin N Am 47 (2014) 135–146
http://dx.doi.org/10.1016/j.otc.2013.08.014
0030-6665/14/$ – see front matter © 2014 Elsevier Inc. All rights reserved.

oto.theclinics.com

Abbreviations	
COPD	Chronic obstructive pulmonary disease
ILS	Irritable larynx syndrome
LCT	Laryngeal control therapy
LPR	Laryngopharyngeal reflux disease
OSA	Obstructive sleep apnea
PFT	Pulmonary function testing
PVFMD	Paradoxic vocal fold movement disorder
SLP	Speech language pathologist

visualized glottic closure in direct correlation with the patient's stridor. In current-day practice, patients with much lesser degrees of stridor and vocal fold narrowing are often evaluated, thanks in great part to the increasing recognition of this disorder by the greater medical community. However, there are clearly still gaps in recognition and understanding of PVFMD.

NATURE OF THE PROBLEM

PVFMD is a disorder in which someone with otherwise normal vocal fold motion suffers from intermittent constriction of the vocal folds during respiration, causing dyspnea and the sensation of throat tightness. The presentation often mimics asthma, although it can occur alongside asthma or other pulmonary disease. The cause of PVFMD was thought to be only psychologic for many years, with stress and anxiety as the primary triggers; the current clinical picture is evolving and may be influenced more by medical comorbidities than previously recognized.[3] Husein and colleagues[4] established in 2008 that 70% of their patients with PVFMD had a psychological profile matching, at least in part, that of a conversion disorder. However, 50% of their patients had comorbid conditions such as gastroesophageal reflux disease or asthma, and they were more likely to have these medical conditions than they were to have a psychiatric history.

Stress and anxiety are still recognized as significant triggers for many patients, but anything that irritates the vocal folds can make paradoxic movement more likely.[3,5–7] There is a well-established link to laryngopharyngeal reflux (LPR), although evidence on whether its treatment leads to resolution of PVFMD is contradictory.[8–14] Laryngeal edema (associated with reflux complaints in 90%) was found in 72% of patients diagnosed with PVFMD in a recent prospective study.[3] This reflux and edema can trigger mild PVFMD in some and full-blown laryngospasm in others.[10]

Other factors that lead to laryngeal mucosal irritation, such as tobacco abuse, allergic laryngitis, viral illness, and untreated sleep apnea, may trigger episodes of PVFMD and make it more difficult to treat.[5,6] Rhinosinusitis and the resulting postnasal drip can directly cause irritation of the vocal folds; however, inflammation may also result indirectly from the release of inflammatory mediators, as described in the "One Airway" theory.[15] Other respiratory tract irritants such as inhaled chemicals, smoke, or gases have long been recognized as prominent triggers in PVFMD as well.[12,16–18] Understanding of the irritable larynx syndrome (ILS), as described by Morrison and colleagues[7] in 1999, is crucial to a full understanding of PVFMD. PVFMD may, in fact, represent a subset of ILS in many cases.[3,5,6]

At the more severe end of this spectrum of vocal fold irritability is laryngeal sensory neuropathy, in which a generalized laryngeal hyperresponsiveness develops after an initial inflammatory insult (such as a viral illness, trauma, or surgery in the neck). Even after controlling for factors such as reflux or allergic inflammation, the patient remains hypersensitive; chronic cough is often present as well.[5] The overlap between PVFMD and laryngeal sensory neuropathy should be recognized, particularly when someone is not responding well to laryngeal control therapy (LCT) alone.

Distinction between PVFMD and the spectrum of vocal cord paresis, paralysis, or synkinesis is crucial. Patients with PVFMD do not have any deficit in vocal fold mobility; full abduction must be seen at some point during the examination to differentiate it from bilateral vocal fold paralysis or paresis. Failure to do so could lead to respiratory embarrassment. Another crucial responsibility of the otolaryngologist, particularly when stridor is present, is ruling out subglottic or tracheal stenosis as the cause of dyspnea.

TERMINOLOGY

The nomenclature associated with PVFMD is confusing; it is also generally unimportant. A shift away from the term "Vocal Cord Dysfunction" has occurred primarily because of confusion with pathologic abnormalities causing dysphonia rather than dyspnea. Laryngologists may receive referrals for "vocal cord dysfunction" when a patient has a lesion of the vocal fold or a vocal fold paralysis, a very different entity from "Vocal Cord Dysfunction," in which there is typically no dysphonia and necessarily no impairment of nerve function or vocal fold mobility. (It should be noted that some authors would disagree that dysphonia is not part of the clinical picture of PVFMD.[19,20])

There is some argument that because a small amount of adduction normally occurs with expiration, the term "paradoxic" is not appropriate when constriction is limited to expiration.[21,22] However, it would be argued that a constriction greater than 50% on either inspiration or expiration is not normal and is paradoxic to the open airway configuration needed for comfortable respiration.

EPIDEMIOLOGY

PVFMD is likely widely underdiagnosed, particularly in rural primary care settings in which asthma not responding to typical treatments is simply assumed to be poorly-controlled. A study of 52 school-age children with suspected poorly controlled asthma found that only 15% actually met criteria for asthma, but 27% were found to have PVFMD.[23] PVFMD has been found to be present at rates of up to 40% among patients with refractory or exercise-induced dyspnea.[19,23–25] Studies focusing specifically on elite athletes and military personnel have been carried out, making it clear that these populations are very much prone to PVFMD as well.[26–28] Another study showed that 20% of female patients undergoing flexible laryngoscopy for any reason were found to have some degree of PVFMD.[29]

There is also the question of whether PVFMD is actually overdiagnosed in some centers. As practitioners in a high-volume laryngology practice often referred to as the "VCD Clinic" within our medical center, we have raised this question ourselves. We now receive referrals for PVFMD evaluations on patients with significant underlying pulmonary disease, such as moderate to severe chronic obstructive pulmonary disease (COPD), but with dyspnea out of proportion to the results of their pulmonary testing. We at first questioned the utility of testing in these patients; glottic constriction on exhalation has been shown in multiple studies to be part of the clinical picture of obstructive pulmonary disease.[25,30–33] However, we are finding that if we see clear improvement of vocal fold abduction with use of the breathing techniques, LCT can help some of these patients decrease the frequency or severity of their dyspnea and medication use. Studies are desperately needed on efficacy of therapy in this group and are underway at the author's institution.

Undiagnosed PVFMD has been shown to lead to immense health care costs.[19,34,35] There are multiple reports of unnecessary intubations and even tracheostomies performed in cases of undiagnosed PVFMD.[36,37] A retrospective case-control study showed that, before their diagnosis, patients with PVFMD had higher utilization of health care than those with moderate persistent asthma.[35] Research is currently underway at the author's institution to study whether asthma medication use decreases after the diagnosis of PVFMD is made.

DIAGNOSIS AND CLINICAL FINDINGS: HISTORY

There are several symptoms and elements of the history that are characteristic of PVFMD (**Box 1**). These elements include a feeling of tightness in the neck or throat, more difficulty getting air in than out, inconsistent or failed response to inhalers, and symptoms that are precipitated by anxiety, strong emotion, odors, changes in humidity or temperature, and exposure to chemicals.[3,7] Dyspnea tends to come on more quickly with PVFMD than with asthma. It also tends to resolve more quickly with rest, rather than becoming most severe after cessation of activity, as in exercise-induced bronchoconstriction.[38,39] In elite athletes particularly, the dyspnea may be provoked only by high-intensity exercise rather than with long, lower-intensity workouts. Patients will often note "wheezing," but on detailed questioning actually describe noisy breathing more on inspiration than expiration. A choking sensation has been found to be more predictive of PVFMD than of exercise-induced bronchoconstriction.[40] It is not uncommon for patients to have breathing "tricks" that they have tried on their own before presentation, often with some success.

In patients who ultimately are diagnosed with both asthma and PVFMD, there is often a distinction between episodes of dyspnea provoked by asthma and those related to PVFMD. Keeping in mind how commonly the two exist together, it is important not to discount the possibility of PVFMD when the patient reports some episodes that respond quickly to albuterol use. These same patients, on detailed questioning, will often say that they can tell the difference between the two even before they unsuccessfully try their inhaler.

DIAGNOSIS AND CLINICAL FINDINGS: PHYSICAL EXAMINATION

Physical examination findings, apart from those found on laryngoscopy (**Box 2**), are nonspecific in PVFMD. The absence of a true end-expiratory wheeze supports the

---

Box 1
History associated with PVFMD

Tightness in neck rather than chest

More difficulty getting air in than out

Symptoms brought on by exertion

Events associated with stress or strong emotions

Events triggered by strong odors, perfumes, or chemicals

Rapid onset of dyspnea

Noisy breathing (usually on inhalation)

Poor or inconsistent response to inhalers

History of negative asthma workup

Box 2

Laryngoscopic findings that support PVFMD

- Severe vocal cord constriction during respiration that corresponds temporally to audible stridor

- Posterior glottic chink during respiration (severe vocal cord adduction with only a small opening posteriorly)

- Greater than 50% narrowing of the glottis occurring at least twice following each of these tasks: breath-holding, counting out loud to 10 on one breath, counting out loud as high as possible during one breath, sustaining an "ee" as long as possible on one breath

- Narrowing of the glottis of greater than 50% occurring during "easy breathing"

- Increased narrowing of the glottis after presentation of strong odors or exertion

- Improvement in vocal fold abduction with use of LCT techniques

Laryngoscopic findings that do not support PVFMD

- Audible stridor heard during full vocal fold abduction

- Constant narrowing on exhalation that worsens with LCT techniques (often seen in COPD patients)

- Failure to fully abduct vocal folds at any point during examination (could indicate a bilateral vocal fold paresis or paralysis)

---

diagnosis, as does the presence of stridor loudest at the neck in the absence of subglottic or tracheal stenosis.

DIAGNOSIS AND CLINICAL FINDINGS: DIAGNOSTIC MODALITIES

Diagnosis of PVFMD requires a flexible laryngoscopic examination, during which the movement of the vocal folds is observed during quiet breathing, after provocative techniques, and again after performance of laryngeal control techniques. This flexible laryngoscopic examination must be performed to confirm the presence of PVFMD, as well as to assess which breathing techniques are most beneficial. It is also absolutely crucial in ruling out actual paralysis, in addition to excluding other pathologic abnormality. The rate of coexistent laryngeal lesions in PVFMD patients has been shown to be as high as 33%.[11,26] Subglottic or tracheal stenosis must also be ruled out. In patients with marked stridor or risk factors for stenosis, lidocaine is often dripped onto the vocal folds and office tracheobronchoscopy performed at the time of their initial evaluation, if imaging of the trachea has not been previously obtained.

Topical decongestant and lidocaine are applied to the nasal cavity before the examination, because it has been shown not to affect vocal fold movement and prevents some of the false positives resulting from poor scope tolerance.[41] Vocal fold movement during respiration in patients without PVFMD typically shows wide abduction with inspiration and slight narrowing with exhalation. Patients with PVFMD show narrowing on inspiration and/or a more marked narrowing on exhalation.[36,39,42–48] The latter is more often seen when the patient is not acutely symptomatic. In some cases the patient will suspend breathing between inhalation and exhalation, with a narrowed glottis. In severe cases of inspiratory narrowing, the "posterior glottic chink" described by Christopher and colleagues[36] in 1983 is seen. Most patients with PVFMD will demonstrate a degree of narrowing even at rest, particularly following the provocative exercises (breath-holding with strong Valsalva, counting out loud as long as possible on a single breath).[13,19,49] If they do not, various strong odors are presented during the laryngoscopic examination (choosing those that are most bothersome to the patient) or the patient is taken to an exertion room where they run on a treadmill as their heart rate and oxygen saturation are monitored. The flexible laryngoscopy is then repeated immediately after the patient reaches the point of feeling dyspneic (**Box 3**). It is rare to get absolutely no narrowing after provocative exercises and attempts to replicate the patient's particular triggers.[49] However, in certain high-risk groups such as young athletes or adults with absolutely no comorbid pulmonary disease, the diagnosis is still suspected even after laryngoscopy does not demonstrate narrowing.[27] It is one of the challenges of diagnosing this disorder that the situation or sport that induces the problem (ie, skiing or swimming) cannot always be replicated. In this setting, a trial of LCT is performed and the flexible laryngoscopy is repeated during therapy (particularly if biofeedback is used as a therapeutic technique) to see if this represents a sampling error. If the patient thinks the breathing techniques are helping him or her, a full course of therapy is continued.

There are numerous diagnostic adjuncts for evaluating PVFMD described in the literature. Besides the laryngoscopic examination described above, the most useful testing is that done by the referring pulmonologist or primary care practitioner. Normal

---

Box 3
Ohio State University protocol for initial laryngoscopic examination in diagnostic evaluation of PVFMD

- Topical lidocaine/Afrin mix is applied to nasal cavities before examination
- Flexible scope is passed via the nasal cavity to observe respiration at rest
- Patient directed to breathe normally so that their typical breathing pattern may be observed
- Patient directed to hold his or her breath for 5 seconds then "let it go"
- Patient directed to count 1 to 10 on one breath
- Patient directed to hold an "ee" or to count out loud as long as he or she can on one breath
- If constriction is observed during normal respiration or following any of the tasks above, the SLP will direct the patient in various therapeutic breathing techniques while the scope is still in place to discover what achieves full abduction. If the LCT techniques worked, they will be enrolled in LCT. Their examination will end here.
- If constriction is not noted and odors are a reported trigger, the patient will be instructed to breathe in strong odors from containers of scents held in front of the patient. These scents include cleaning agents, perfumes, and potpourri. If a reaction is noted, the SLP will direct the patient in various therapeutic breathing techniques while the scope is still in place to discover what achieves full abduction. If the LCT techniques worked, they will be enrolled in LCT. Their examination will end here.
- When a patient does not exhibit constriction with strong odors or during normal respiration, the scope will be removed but the evaluation will not end. The patient will be directed to participate in exertional activities until symptomatic or until heart rate is significantly elevated (treadmill, riding a stationary bike, climbing stairs, jumping jacks). The laryngoscopic examination will then be repeated immediately to observe for glottic narrowing during the presence of symptoms. The SLP will direct the patient in various therapeutic breathing techniques while the scope is still in place to discover what achieves full abduction. If the breathing techniques worked, they will be enrolled in LCT. Their examination will end here.
- If narrowing has still not been observed by this point, the patient's symptoms, history, and overall clinical picture are assessed to determine whether a trial of LCT is appropriate.

pulmonary function testing (PFT), inspiratory limb flattening on flow volume loop, or increased symptoms after methacholine challenge (without good response to bronchodilator) all support the diagnosis of PVFMD.[19,25,28,40,44,50–53]

Pulmonary testing is typically done prior to referral for PVFMD. Pulmonary testing is important, because the presence of PVFMD does not exclude coexistent pulmonary disease and should not lead to complacency on the part of the physician working up the patient's dyspnea. Conversely, the presence of abnormal pulmonary testing also does not rule out PVFMD. It is crucial to understand that, in our experience, even patients with moderately severe underlying pulmonary disease can occasionally benefit from LCT, if constriction is present and if the laryngeal control techniques are shown to improve vocal fold abduction during the initial diagnostic laryngoscopy. Occasionally (although rarely) the breathing techniques can actually make the sensation of dyspnea worse; this seems most common in COPD patients and can be predicted when a pattern of consistent (rather than intermittent) glottic narrowing on exhalation is seen.[25,30–33] As mentioned above, however, the use of LCT for patients with moderately severe underlying lung disease has not been well studied to this point.

MANAGEMENT GOALS

The foremost goal of management is subjective improvement in dyspnea. Associated goals include resumption of athletic or social events that were previously avoided, means of managing future exacerbations brought on by illness or stress, cessation of unnecessary asthma medication use, and avoidance of Emergency Department visits or missed work or school.

TREATMENT: LCT WITH A SPEECH LANGUAGE PATHOLOGIST

There is no standard pharmacologic management of PVFMD besides that used to control comorbid conditions. The cornerstone of treatment of PVFMD is LCT, also called respiratory retraining therapy, performed by a licensed speech language pathologist (SLP). It has been shown to be effective in up to 95% of patients.[26,54] A lengthy description of specific therapy techniques is beyond the scope of the article; **Box 4** describes basic principles. In treating patients who have failed LCT performed elsewhere, the addition of desensitization and biofeedback has been found to be helpful if not previously done; old therapy records can be reviewed to help decide between a repeat course of therapy versus a different diagnostic path altogether.[55] It is also

---

Box 4
Brief instruction in LCT techniques

- Low abdominal breathing with pressurized breaths
- Breath should be pressurized through a point of constriction at the nose or lips
- Lips should be rounded and the breath noisy
- Envision "shooting a column of air out" through the lips
- A straw cut in thirds can serve as a prop to teach the proper technique initially, with the patient exhaling through it and blowing a cool, forceful stream of air toward their hand held out in front of them
- Breaths should be performed slowly so as not to hyperventilate
- Patients are instructed to practice techniques a total of 10 minutes a day to reinforce muscle memory and achieve a more abducted vocal fold position over time

important to ensure that the SLP who is treating the patient is comfortable with providing LCT. SLPs are becoming more specialized, just as physicians are, and LCT is not always part of the repertoire of, for example, a hospital-based SLP who typically works to rehabilitate stroke patients.

TREATMENT: ADDRESSING UNDERLYING PSYCHIATRIC ISSUES

The psychologic underpinnings of PVFMD cannot be overlooked. Besides the studies discussed above that link PVFMD to conversion disorder, there is also literature demonstrating a high rate of psychiatric diagnoses and history of sexual abuse in these patients.[19,25,56,57] Although these studies may not be representative of the population at a high-volume PVFMD clinic within a medical system that widely recognizes its prevalence, they do point out how important it is to screen these patients for undiagnosed underlying psychiatric issues or possible abuse, particularly when not responding well to therapy or control of medical comorbidities. Counseling and even pharmacologic management of anxiety can be an important adjunct in these cases.

TREATMENT: ELITE ATHLETES

Elite athletes with PVFMD have different characteristics and may require a different treatment approach than the general population with PVFMD. There is a lower rate of psychiatric pathology in elite athletes, as demonstrated by the recent review by Chiang and colleagues.[26] They also have lower rates of coexistent reflux. They tend to have primarily exertion-induced symptoms and may require therapy sessions performed "on site" (ie, on the football field, tennis court, or track) to identify subtle provoking factors and to achieve the necessary degree of exertion needed to carry out adequate desensitization.

TREATMENT: INVESTIGATIONAL THERAPIES

Inhaled anticholinergic was shown to prevent PVFMD triggered by exertion when used before onset of activity in a very small retrospective study.[58] Continuous positive airway pressure has been shown to relieve expiratory constriction in case reports,[31] and an investigational mask that functions as a one-way "inspiratory valve" was developed to decrease the rate of inspiratory airflow, reducing stridor and perhaps breaking the spiral of anxiety and distress that patients feel when they hear their own noisy breathing.[59] For acute or severe cases, benzodiazepines, heliox, and even laryngeal botox have been used with some benefit.[51,60,61]

TREATMENT: COMORBID CONDITIONS

Managing reflux, allergies, sinus disease, and extreme dryness is crucial and often leads to the prescription of medications during the evaluation of PVFMD. Untreated obstructive sleep apnea (OSA) also seems to contribute to the development of PVFMD, although more research must be done in this area. Asthma often coexists with PVFMD, but PVFMD can also be misdiagnosed as asthma. In the latter situation, patients are often on unnecessary inhalers that can actually worsen the PVFMD. If coexistent asthma has been ruled out, the importance of stopping steroid and β-agonist inhalers is strongly emphasized; this eliminates the risk for fungal laryngitis, decreases dryness, and generally reduces the degree of laryngeal irritation, making the PVFMD easier to treat.

TREATMENT: SELF-MANAGEMENT STRATEGIES

Some insurance providers do not cover LCT or place limits on the amount of therapy; in these situations it is helpful to show patients some simple techniques they can try on their own (see **Box 4**). In all cases patients are shown the video of their laryngoscopy, which is used to point out the vocal fold narrowing and help them better understand the condition. They are also educated in general vocal hygiene and in identifying and avoiding triggers and common vocal fold irritants. The particular breathing techniques that were most helpful to them during the laryngoscopic exam are redemonstrated. Many patients seem to benefit from simply understanding the cause of their dyspneic episodes, even if they are not able to go through a full course of treatment.

TREATMENT: RECURRENCE

Patients should be warned that recurrence is frequent at times of illness or flare in allergy or reflux symptoms. To minimize this, patients are encouraged to practice the breathing techniques even when asymptomatic to develop the "muscle memory" that will keep the glottis more widely abducted during respiration. In addition to control of comorbid conditions, a "refresher session" of LCT may be helpful, along with desensitization and biofeedback if not previously done. However, if symptoms that were previously controlled do not improve with therapy, focus should then shift to look for other underlying factors such as new or worsened pulmonary disease, cardiac problems, or airway stenosis.

SUMMARY

PVFMD is typically a very treatable cause of dyspnea, so long as it is identified. However, it is also a multifactorial disease, and treatment must be tailored to the individual patient and his or her particular comorbid conditions. Failure to recognize PVFMD can lead to immense health care costs. Important challenges include (1) ensuring PVFMD is considered when a pulmonary workup is negative or does not fully explain the dyspnea, and (2) identifying SLPs who are experienced in the treatment of PVFMD. Treating comorbidities such as reflux disease, allergies, asthma, and psychiatric illness remain important, and ruling out underlying vocal fold paralysis or airway stenosis is crucial.

REFERENCES

1. Dunglison RD. The practice of medicine. Philadelphia: Lea and Blanchard; 1842. p. 257–8.
2. Mackenzie M. Use of laryngoscopy in disease of the throat. Philadelphia: Lindsey and Blackeston; 1869. p. 246–50.
3. Forrest LA, Husein T, Husein O. Paradoxical vocal cord motion: classification and treatment. Laryngoscope 2012;122(4):844–53.
4. Husein OF, Husein TN, Gardner R, et al. Formal psychological testing in patients with paradoxical vocal fold dysfunction. Laryngoscope 2008;118(4):740–7.
5. Ayres JG, Gabbott PL. Vocal cord dysfunction and laryngeal hyperresponsiveness: a function of altered autonomic balance? Thorax 2002;57:284–5.
6. Bucca C, Rolla G, Brussino L, et al. Are asthma-like symptoms due to bronchial or extrathoracic airway dysfunction? Lancet 1995;346:791–5.
7. Morrison M, Rammage L, Emami AJ. The irritable larynx syndrome. J Voice 1999;13(3):447–55.

8. Denoyelle F, Garabedian EN, Roger G, et al. Laryngeal dyskinesias as a cause of stridor in infants. Arch Otolaryngol Head Neck Surg 1996;122:612–6.

9. Koufman JA. Paradoxical vocal fold movement. Voice 1994;3:49–53, 70–1.

10. Loughlin CJ, Koufman JA, Averill DB, et al. Acid induced laryngospasm in a canine model. Laryngoscope 1996;106:1506–9.

11. Patel NJ, Jorgensen C, Kuhn J, et al. Concurrent laryngeal abnormalities in patients with paradoxical vocal fold dysfunction. Otolaryngol Head Neck Surg 2004;130:686–9.

12. Perkner JJ, Fennelly KP, Balkisson R, et al. Irritant associated vocal cord dysfunction. J Occup Environ Med 1998;40:136–43.

13. Powell DM, Karanfilov BI, Beechler KB, et al. Paradoxical vocal cord dysfunction in juveniles. Arch Otolaryngol Head Neck Surg 2000;126:29–34.

14. Maschka DA, Bauman NM, McCray PB, et al. A classification scheme for paradoxical vocal cord motion. Laryngoscope 1997;107:1429–35.

15. Grossman J. One airway, one disease. Chest 1997;111(Suppl 2):11S–6S.

16. Andrianopoulos MV, Gallivan GJ, Gallivan KH. PVCM, PVCD, EPL and irritable larynx syndrome: what are we talking about and how do we treat it? J Voice 2000;14:607–18.

17. Bhargava S, Panitch HB, Allen JL. Chlorine induced paradoxical vocal cord dysfunction. Chest 2000;118:2955S–6S.

18. Galdi E, Perfetti L, Pagella F, et al. Irritant vocal cord dysfunction at first misdiagnosed as reactive airway dysfunction syndrome. Scand J Work Environ Health 2005;31:224–6.

19. Newman KB, Mason UG, Schmaling KB. Clinical features of vocal cord dysfunction. Am J Respir Crit Care Med 1995;152:1382–6.

20. Parsons JP, Benninger C, Hawley MP, et al. Vocal cord dysfunction: beyond severe asthma. Respir Med 2010;104(4):504–9.

21. Christopher KL, Morris MJ. Vocal cord dysfunction, paradoxic vocal fold motion, or laryngomalacia? Our understanding requires an interdisciplinary approach [review]. Otolaryngol Clin North Am 2010;43(1):43–66. http://dx.doi.org/10.1016/j.otc.2009.12.002, viii.

22. Christopher KL. Understanding vocal cord dysfunction. A step in the right direction with a long road ahead. Chest 2006;129:842–3.

23. Sear M, Wensley D, West N. How accurate is the diagnosis of exercise-induced asthma among Vancouver school children? Arch Dis Child 2005;90:898–902.

24. Kenn K, Willer G, Bizer C, et al. Prevalence of vocal cord dysfunction in patient with dyspnoea. First prospective clinical study. Am J Respir Crit Care Med 1997;155:A965.

25. Newman KB, Dubester SN. Vocal cord dysfunction. Masquerader of asthma. Semin Respir Crit Care Med 1994;15:161–7.

26. Chiang T, Marcinow AM, DeSilva BW, et al. Exercise-induced paradoxical vocal fold motion disorder: diagnosis and management. Laryngoscope 2012;123:727–31.

27. Hanks CD, Parsons J, Benninger C, et al. Etiology of dyspnea in elite and recreational athletes. Phys Sportsmed 2012;40(2):28–33.

28. Morris MJ, Deal LE, Bean DR, et al. Vocal cord dysfunction in patients with dyspnea. Chest 1999;116:1676–82.

29. O'Connell MA, Sklarew PR, Goodman DL. Spectrum of presentation of paradoxical vocal cord motion in ambulatory patients. Ann Allergy Asthma Immunol 1995;74:341–4.

30. Collett PW, Brancatisano T, Engel LA. Changes in the glottis aperture during bronchial asthma. Am Rev Respir Dis 1983;128(4):719–23.
31. Goldman J, Muers M. Vocal cord dysfunction and wheezing. Thorax 1991;46: 401–4.
32. Higenbottam T. Narrowing of the glottis opening in humans associated with experimentally induced bronchoconstriction. J Apply Physiol 1980;49(3): 403–7.
33. Higenbottam T, Payne J. Glottis narrowing in lung disease. Am Rev Respir Dis 1982;125(6):746–50.
34. Cohen SM, Belluci E. Health utilization among patients with vocal cord dysfunction. Nurs Forum 2011;46(3):177–85.
35. Mikita J, Parker J. High levels of medical utilization by ambulatory patients with vocal cord dysfunction as compared to age and gender matched asthmatics. Chest 2006;129:905–8.
36. Christopher KL, Wood RP, Eckert C, et al. Vocal cord dysfunction presenting as asthma. N Engl J Med 1983;308:1566–70.
37. Patterson R, Schatz M, Horton M. Munchausen's stridor: non-organic laryngeal obstruction. Clin Allergy 1974;4(3):307–10.
38. Anderson SD, Silverman M, Konig P, et al. Exercise induced asthma. Br J Dis Chest 1975;69:1–39.
39. Rundell KW, Spiering BA. Inspiratory stridor in elite athletes. Chest 2003;123(2): 468–74.
40. Guss J, Mirza N. Methacholine challenge testing in the diagnosis of paradoxical vocal fold motion. Laryngoscope 2006;116(9):1558–61.
41. Pitchenik AE. Functional laryngeal obstruction relived by panting. Chest 1991; 100:1465–7.
42. Alpert SE, Dearborn DG, Kercsmar CM. On vocal cord dysfunction in wheezy children. Pediatr Pulmonol 1991;10:142–3.
43. Altman KW, Mirza N, Ruiz C, et al. Paradoxical cord fold motion: presentation and treatment options. J Voice 2000;14:99–103.
44. Bahrainwala AH, Simon MR, Harrison DD, et al. Atypical expiratory flow volume curve in an asthmatic patient with vocal cord dysfunction. Ann Allergy Asthma Immunol 2001;86(4):438–43.
45. Cohen JI. Clinical conferences at the Johns Hopkins Hospital. Upper airway obstruction in asthma. Johns Hopkins Med J 1980;147(6):233–7.
46. Kivity S, Bibi H, Schwarz Y, et al. Variable vocal cord dysfunction presenting as wheezing and exercise induced asthma. J Asthma 1986;23:241–4.
47. Rothe TB, Karrer W. Therapy-resistent asthma: causes and therapy. Pracis 1995;84(40):1118–24.
48. Heimdal JH, Roskund OD, Halvorsen T, et al. Continuous laryngoscopic exercise test: a method for visualizing laryngeal dysfunction during exercise. Laryngoscope 2006;116:52–7.
49. Treole L, Trudeau MD, Forrest LA. Endoscopic and stroboscopic description of adults with paradoxical vocal fold dysfunction. J Voice 1999;13:143–52.
50. Brown IG, Zamel N, Hoffstein V. Pharyngeal and glottic changes following methacholine challenge in normal subjects. Bull Eur Physiopathol Respir 1986;22: 251–6.
51. Morris MJ, Allan PF, Perkins PJ. Vocal cord dysfunction, aetiologies and treatment. Clin Pulm Med 2006;13:73–86.
52. Perkins PJ, Morris MJ. Vocal cord dysfunction induced by methacholine challenge testing. Chest 2002;122:1988–93.

53. Vlahakis NE, Patel AM, Maragos NE, et al. Diagnosis of vocal cord dysfunction: the utility of spirometry and plethysmography. Chest 2002;122(6):2246–9.
54. Sullivan MD, Heywood BM, Beukelman DR. A treatment for vocal cord dysfunction in female athletes: an outcome study. Laryngoscope 2001;111:1751–5.
55. Nahimas J, Tansey M, Karetzky MS. Asthmatic extrathoracic upper airway obstruction: laryngeal dyskinesis. N J Med 1994;91:616–20.
56. Freedman MR, Rosenberg SJ, Schmaling KB. Childhood sexual abuse in patients with paradoxical vocal fold dysfunction. J Nerv Ment Dis 1991;179:295–8.
57. Leo RJ, Konakanchi R. Psychogenic respiratory distress a case of paradoxical vocal cord dysfunction and literature review. Prim Care Companion J Clin Psychiatry 1999;1:439–46.
58. Doshi DR, Weinberger MM. Long-term outcome of vocal cord dysfunction. Ann Allergy Asthma Immunol 2006;96:794–9.
59. Archer GJ, Hoyle JK, Cluskey AM, et al. Inspiratory vocal cord dysfunction, a new approach in treatment. Eur Respir J 2000;15:617–8.
60. Maillard I, Schweizer V, Broccard A, et al. Use of botulinum toxin type A to avoid tracheal intubation or tracheostomy in severe paradoxical vocal cord movement. Chest 2000;118:874–7.
61. Weir M. Vocal cord dysfunction mimics asthma and may respond to heliox. Clin Pediatr 2002;41:37–41.

Other Asthma Considerations

Patrick R. Aguilar, MD[a], Evan S. Walgama, MD[b],
Matthew W. Ryan, MD[b],*

KEYWORDS

- Asthma • Aspirin-exacerbated respiratory disease • Foreign body aspiration
- Cough-variant asthma • Work-related asthma • Hypersensitivity pneumonitis
- Churg-Strauss • Allergic bronchopulmonary aspergillosis

KEY POINTS

- Patients with difficult-to-treat asthma should be evaluated for alternative diagnoses.
- Aspirin-exacerbated respiratory disease consists of the triad of sinonasal polyposis, bronchial asthma, and aspirin intolerance. Diagnosis is confirmed by oral aspirin challenge. Aspirin desensitization may improve otherwise difficult-to-control sinusitis and asthma in these patients.
- Foreign-body aspiration is an important mimicker of asthma in children. Rigid bronchoscopy can secure the diagnosis and early foreign-body removal will prevent long-term complications.
- Patients with nonasthmatic eosinophilic bronchitis have chronic cough, sputum eosinophilia, and absent bronchial hyper-reactivity on spirometry. Inhaled-corticosteroids therapy may be effective.
- Work-related asthma is a complex syndrome involving potential inducers or exacerbators of bronchoconstriction that relate to occupational exposure. Among patients with difficult-to-treat asthma, historical assessment should include a review of workplace exposures and symptomatic changes with work avoidance.
- Hypersensitivity pneumonitis represents a distinct pathophysiologic entity involving alveolar lymphocytosis. Patients with exposure-related symptoms may benefit from altered therapy based on proper delineation of pathophysiologic mechanism of disease.
- Churg-Strauss syndrome is a progressive constellation of rhinosinusitis, nasal polyposis, asthma, vasculitis, and peripheral neuropathy. Initiation of therapy early in disease course can alter progression and slow the development of visceral vasculitic damage.
- Allergic bronchopulmonary aspergillosis can complicate the management of asthma. Asthma clinicians should maintain a low threshold of suspicion to prompt close investigation for this process in patients with difficult-to-treat asthma, fevers, weight loss, or expectoration of mucus plugs.

Financial Disclosures: Dr M.W. Ryan has served on advisory boards for Teva and Sunovion, and as a promotional speaker for Sunovion.
Conflict of Interest: None.
[a] Department of Internal Medicine, Washington University, 660 Euclid, PO Box 8052, St. Louis, MO 63110, USA; [b] Department of Otolaryngology-Head and Neck Surgery, University of Texas Southwestern Medical Center, 5323 Harry Hines Boulevard, Dallas, TX 75390-9035, USA
* Corresponding author.
E-mail address: matthew.ryan@utsouthwestern.edu

Otolaryngol Clin N Am 47 (2014) 147–160
http://dx.doi.org/10.1016/j.otc.2013.08.015
0030-6665/14/$ – see front matter © 2014 Elsevier Inc. All rights reserved.

INTRODUCTION

Asthma is a heterogeneous syndrome of cough, wheeze, dyspnea, and chest tightness that affects approximately 300 million individuals worldwide. Pathologically, airways are characterized by chronic inflammation and diminished bronchial diameter. Physiologically, spirometry demonstrates a degree of reversible airflow obstruction typically responsive to bronchodilators. Although these physiologic and pathologic distinctions contribute to the definition of asthma, the clinical symptoms of this syndrome provide practitioners little help in arriving at a specific diagnosis. Given the prevalence of asthma and the relative paucity of so-called asthma mimickers, the common constellation of cough, wheeze, dyspnea, and chest tightness usually signifies underlying asthma. However, in a subset of patients, these symptoms may represent a different underlying disease process with variable responsiveness to classic asthma therapies. In these patients, disease may progress while practitioners attempt conventional therapy. Some types of asthma may require alternative approaches to relieve symptoms successfully.

Although the aim of this article is to clarify the differential diagnosis of asthma to the otolaryngologist, the list of potential mimickers is broad (**Box 1**). Patients with bronchial wall edema from congestive heart failure may have concomitant wheezing and dyspnea unrelated to airway inflammation, whereas obese patients may experience symptoms consistent with asthma without any significant bronchial diameter-related reduction in airflow. Similarly, there are a wide array of causes that may produce chronic wheezing, cough, and shortness of breath in any particular patient. This article addresses some of the more common medical and surgical processes that may be encountered in the practice of asthma management. For each diagnosis, awareness of the potential will increase the practitioner's likelihood of considering (and evaluating for) an alternative pathologic condition in an at-risk patient.

Box 1
Differential diagnosis of asthma

Acute bronchitis

Allergic bronchopulmonary aspergillosis

Chronic obstructive pulmonary disease

Churg-Strauss syndrome

Congestive heart failure

Foreign body aspiration

Hypersensitivity pneumonitis

Laryngopharyngeal reflux

Nonasthmatic eosinophilic bronchitis

Obesity

Tracheal or bronchial stenosis

Vascular ring

Vocal cord dysfunction

Work-related asthma

ASPIRIN-EXACERBATED RESPIRATORY DISEASE

Otolarygologists are familiar with Samter's triad, in which patients present with recalcitrant sinonasal polyposis, aspirin sensitivity, and asthma. This eponymous entity is now more commonly called aspirin-exacerbated respiratory disease (AERD) or aspirin-induced asthma. The hallmark of the disease is an adverse response to ingestion of aspirin or nonsteroidal antiinflammatory drugs (NSAIDs), after which patients can experience exacerbations of both upper and lower airway disease. The rhinosinusitis experienced by patients with AERD is severe compared with other subtypes of chronic rhinosinusitis and may be refractory to standard medical and surgical therapies.[1]

Mucosal inflammation in AERD is related to disordered metabolism of arachidonic acid, which is metabolized by the cyclooxygenase (COX) pathway to yield prostaglandins or by the lipoxygenase pathway to yield cysteinyl leukotrienes. Aspirin and other NSAIDs block the COX pathway, shunting metabolism away from antiinflammatory prostaglandins toward proinflammatory cysteinyl leukotrienes.[2] Cysteinyl leukotrienes are important mediators in the pathophysiology of asthma and, possibly, in the development of sinonasal polyposis in asthmatics. Patients with AERD have elevated levels of urinary cysteinyl leukotrienes compared with aspirin-tolerant asthmatics, as do aspirin-tolerant asthmatics with sinonasal polyposis compared with asthmatics without sinonasal disease.[3]

Patients with AERD commonly develop symptoms in early adulthood.[4,5] They may report an upper respiratory infection that "never went away," or an exposure to a COX-1 inhibitor that marked the beginning of their symptoms. Nearly all patients with AERD have sinonasal symptoms, followed by adult-onset asthma.[4]

Patients with suspected AERD are confirmed by an oral aspirin challenge. Protocols exist that typically take 2 to 3 days of outpatient supervision to complete.[6] In a review of 300 patients referred to a tertiary center for a history of adverse reaction to aspirin-related drugs, 85% had a positive reaction to an oral aspirin provocation.[5] Aspirin provocation followed by desensitization differs from standard immunotherapy in that a reaction is expected to occur. A reaction may include naso-ocular symptoms, lower airway reactivity measured by forced expiratory volume in 1 second (FEV_1), laryngospasm, anaphylactoid reaction, or some combination of these. After a positive oral challenge, the patient can be treated either by avoidance of all COX-1 inhibitors or by desensitization, which involves continued escalation of the dose of aspirin into the therapeutic range, followed by continuous aspirin therapy.[6]

Continuous aspirin therapy in patients with AERD results in decreased bronchial reactivity, decreased dependence on topical steroids and albuterol, and improvement in nasal symptoms.[7,8] McMains and Kountakis[9] performed a retrospective review of AERD patients undergoing endoscopic sinus surgery and showed that eight out of ten patients who did not received aspirin desensitization required revision sinus surgery, whereas no patients receiving aspirin therapy required revision in the 2-year follow-up period. Initiation of aspirin desensitization is typically performed 4 weeks following endoscopic sinus surgery.

After sinus surgery, AERD patients may benefit from treatment with a leukotriene-modifying drug combined with a topical nasal steroid.[2] Leukotriene-modifying drugs include those that block the leukotriene receptor, currently montelukast and zafirlukast, as well as zileuton, which block the 5-lipooygenase enzyme further upstream. These drugs should be continued if the patient is to undergo aspirin oral challenge and desensitization.[10]

Asthma in patients with AERD responds to traditional asthma therapies but can be difficult to control. The typical patient with AERD will require both a topical corticosteroid and a leukotriene-modifying drug for control of their asthma. Concomitant atopic disease should not be ignored and may be treated with allergen avoidance, antihistamines, anti-IgE therapy, or immunotherapy as indicated.

FOREIGN-BODY ASPIRATION

In children, foreign-body aspiration can present with symptoms of bronchial asthma. Children usually present after a coughing or choking spell.[11] Children of any age may present, though typically they are younger than 2 years of age. Most patients present to emergency rooms soon after suspected aspiration; those presenting to outpatient providers days or weeks after the event may be more easily confused with bronchial asthma. Physical examination may show unilateral decreased breath sounds or wheezing. Other findings may include tachypnea, stridor, coughing, fever, or cyanosis. Chest radiographs may show evidence of air trapping or atelectasis of distal lung parenchyma. However, a high index of suspicion should not be allayed by a normal physical examination and radiographic evaluation because neither of these is sensitive for the detection of airway foreign body in children.[12] Patients in whom foreign-body aspiration is suspected should undergo rigid bronchoscopy for diagnosis and possible removal of the foreign body.

A delay in diagnosis can lead to inappropriate treatments for asthma or pneumonia, and can result in a prolonged hospital stay compared with a prompt diagnosis resulting in interventional bronchoscopy.[11] A significant delay in diagnosis can result in chronic respiratory sequelae including bronchiectasis.[13]

COUGH VARIANT ASTHMA OR NONASTHMATIC EOSINOPHILIC BRONCHITIS

Asthma represents 25% to 29% of cases of chronic cough.[14] Although the typical triad of wheezing, shortness of breath, and chest tightness often accompanies cough in cases of asthma, a subset of patients with asthma will report cough as their predominant (if not only) symptom of concern. This syndrome, termed cough variant asthma (CVA), is associated with mast cell airway infiltration, airway remodeling, and reversible airflow obstruction in a pattern consistent with other forms of asthma.[15]

The workup of chronic cough generally includes measurement of airflow limitation by spirometry. Although some patients with CVA demonstrate abnormalities in their pulmonary function tests, many have essentially normal spirometry. Given the vague nature of an isolated cough in a nonsmoking patient with normal spirometry, diagnosis of CVA requires a high index of suspicion for the diagnosis in this population. Methacholine inhalation challenge will typically demonstrate increased bronchial reactivity, which supports a diagnosis of CVA.[14] However, diagnosis typically requires response to a diagnostic or therapeutic trial of bronchodilators and inhaled corticosteroids. Patients with concerning symptoms should start a trial of therapy consistent with general guideline-based management of asthma.[16] A 14-day course of the leukotriene receptor antagonist zafirlukast was demonstrated to improve subjective cough score in a series of patients with bronchodilator and inhaled-corticosteroid refractory CVA.[17] Therefore, patients with failure of response to bronchodilator and inhaled-corticosteroid therapy should be offered second-line leukotriene-receptor antagonist therapy. In some patients with severe disease, a short course of systemic corticosteroids may be useful as an adjunct to chronic therapy.[18] Treatment should continue in a fashion consistent with guideline-driven asthma therapy. However, even with therapy, up to 30% of patients with CVA eventually progress to classic asthma.[19]

CVA demonstrates a sputum eosinophilia similar to that observed in classic asthma.[20] However, up to 13% of patients with chronic cough present with sputum eosinophilia, chronic cough, and absence of spirometric markers of bronchial hyper-reactivity.[21] This syndrome, known as nonasthmatic eosinophilic bronchitis, represents a constellation of normal spirometry, increased cough, sputum eosinophilia, and absent bronchodilator response.[22] Patients presenting with this symptomatic array should be evaluated for occupational or environmental exposures, and be considered for a trial of inhaled corticosteroids. Inhaled budesonide has resulted in a decrease in sputum eosinophils and cough reflex sensitivity among patients with eosinophilic bronchitis.[23]

The differential diagnosis of chronic cough is broad. Workup should include evaluation for sputum eosinophilia and bronchial hyper-reactivity. Early recognition of the diagnoses of CVA and eosinophilic bronchitis requires disease awareness and a low threshold of suspicion. Such diagnosis may result in earlier administration of appropriate therapy and shorter duration of symptoms.

WORK-RELATED ASTHMA

Work-related asthma (WRA) is a broad term encompassing several circumstances in which asthma symptoms are either triggered or exacerbated by work exposures. Occupational asthma (OA) is a specific subset of bronchial hyper-reactivity associated with variable airflow limitation occurring de novo (or recurring in an asthmatic patient previously in remission) in the setting of a specific agent related to the workplace. This can take the form of an immediate response (ie, reactive airway dysfunction syndrome or irritant-induced OA) that is independent of allergic reaction. In other circumstances, patients may experience progressive bronchoconstriction resulting from development of an allergic response to a workplace substance (ie, sensitizer-induced OA). A separate subset of WRA called work-exacerbated asthma (WEA) is the worsening of pre-existing asthma by work-related noxious exposure (**Box 2**).[24,25]

As the leading occupation-related lung disease in many countries, OA generates a significant amount of interest among employers and managers of workers' compensation funds, and accounts for 9% to 15% of cases of adult asthma.[26] As a result, there is much written about the cause and definition of this syndrome as well as the association between symptoms and work-related exposures. Further confounding the analysis of this complex disease, diagnostic standards are less than optimally homogeneous, particularly given the medico-legal and financial implications of a work-related diagnosis.

Typically, patients present with classic asthma symptoms of shortness of breath, chest tightness, wheezing, and cough that variably improves during periods away from work exposures. Whereas some patients may have improvement in symptoms during their daily time off, many require a more extensive period away from the trigger to induce remission of symptoms. Symptomatic improvement during weekends or on prolonged vacations has approximately 88% to 90% sensitivity for OA.[27] Therefore,

---

Box 2
OA

Sensitizer-induced OA: progressive bronchoconstriction resulting from development of an allergic response to a workplace substance

Irritant-induced OA: immediate bronchoconstriction from direct noxious stimulus by workplace substance

WEA: preexisting asthma symptoms made worse by occupational exposure

when evaluating a patient with asthma, clinicians should inquire about variations in symptoms related to time off. In patients with new onset symptoms, historical review should also include ascertainment of work tasks, specific exposures (with review of material safety data sheets), changes in work processes or work areas, adherence to personnel protection-equipment policies, unusual exposures within 24 hours of symptoms or concomitant sinonasal or conjunctival irritation. Patients should also be asked to describe any history of reactive airway disease to elucidate the potential for WEA. Physical examination should target wheezing, allergic mucosal changes, or dysphonia, though these are all nonspecific findings and do not definitively direct the clinician's focus. Although historical assessment and physical examination are imperative to identify other potentially pathologic causes, only 50% of diagnoses of OA are likely to result from history or examination alone.

Literally hundreds of substances have been associated with WRA. Health workers have been noted to have symptom development with latex gloves, hairdressers have had symptomatic association with persulfates, and plant workers have become progressively ill with exposures to a wide variety of workplace agents.[28] Although specific inhalational challenges may help with objectively documenting bronchial reactivity, initial workup should begin with pulmonary function testing, including bronchodilator responses and nonspecific challenges (either methacholine or histamine), to determine bronchial responsiveness.

If historical information raises suspicion of WRA, patients may be asked to provide data from serial peak expiratory flow rate (PEFR) measured both at and away from work. After training on proper performance of PEFR, patients perform measurements four times daily, ideally for 3 to 4 weeks. This is completed on both workdays and on days off. Optimally, it includes a 2-week period off for comparison to a 2-week period of work. Although there is difficulty in interpreting the significance of variability based on gross analysis of PEFR results, these measurements can be imported into the OASYS system (Occupational Asthma Expert SYStem, Vitalograph, UK) with a computer-driven differential analysis. Variability of greater than 20% to 30% in peak flow measurements as assessed by this software is associated with 78% sensitivity and 92% specificity for OA.[29]

Additionally, physiologic measurements of airway responsiveness can be obtained sequentially after prolonged exposure (eg, the end of a workweek) and a period of prolonged avoidance (eg, a 2-week vacation). This can be accomplished using spirometry with methacholine or histamine challenges. After a week of work, a threefold decline in the concentration of provocative substance necessary to produce a 20% fall in FEV_1 would be additional support for a diagnosis of WRA.[25] Although allergic skin testing can be helpful in the assessment of an IgE response to protein allergens (eg, animal dander), most chemical irritants have not similarly been associated with positive results. Similarly, specific serologic IgE antibodies have been associated with many protein (but few chemical) triggers for asthma. The role of targeted immunologic testing (serologic or skin) has been addressed in several studies but remains unclear. Generally, this battery of tests may help identify specific triggers in some patients with OA symptoms, though it obviously does not exclude untested triggers.[25]

Specific inhalation challenges (SICs) have been described by the US Agency for Healthcare Research and Quality as a "reference standard" for OA.[30] These tests remain cumbersome, fraught with confounding technicalities, and accessible only at a few centers worldwide. Nonetheless, SIC may be a useful adjunct in the diagnosis of WRA in an otherwise unclear case. Alternatively, in a review of 10 patients with WRA, there was notation of a significant increase in median (interquartile range) sputum eosinophils during a 2-week to 4-week period of work when compared with a 2-week period away. This suggests that sputum cell counts may provide yet another clue in the workup of the patient with suspected WRA.[31] In summary, the rational approach to the diagnosis of WRA should include historical assessment of respiratory symptoms, association of symptoms with work exposures, and physiologic assessments of response to work exposure. Although there is no gold standard, these factors can be used in combination to provide support for such a diagnosis.

Of note, occupational exposure-related lung disease may manifest in a variety of ways. Hypersensitivity pneumonitis (HP) may present in similar fashion to OA (see later discussion). However, the underlying pathophysiology of OA remains a type-1 hypersensitivity reaction (prominent IgE response), consistent with other types of asthma. In contradistinction, HP is mediated by T-lymphocytes and it represents a type-4 hypersensitivity reaction. This important difference drives the variability in therapy between two similar phenotypes with similar exposures.

Therapy for WRA is driven by subtype of disease. For all patients, irritant avoidance remains the principal mechanism for improvement in symptoms. However, this is not always easy to achieve, particularly if the diagnosis is unclear. For patients with sensitizer-induced OA, therapy should be avoidance of, or reduction in exposure to, the noxious stimulus responsible for illness. Given that this may not be possible for economic or personal reasons, bronchodilator therapy (to include inhaled corticosteroids and/or β2-agonists) may be applied in the fashion generally prescribed for non-OA. Irritant-induced asthma occurs after a very short latent period and represents an acute response to a respiratory irritant. Therefore, engineering processes and personnel protective equipment is often able to reduce burden to such a degree that symptomatic recurrence is prevented. WEA has some pathophysiologic differences from simple progression of asthma. However, very few studies have been targeted at defining variation in therapy for patients with this syndrome. As a result, management of asthma in conventional fashion with maximal exposure avoidance remains the most prudent course of therapy.[25]

HP

HP is a complex clinical syndrome of nonspecific pulmonary symptomatology resulting from recurrent antigen exposure, IgG activation, and alveolar lymphocytosis with subsequent damage to lung architecture. Known toxic antigens include inhaled mycobacterial, bacterial, fungal, animal protein, and chemical substances (**Table 1**).[32] In a series analyzing rates of occupational lung disease in the United Kingdom between 1992 and 2001, there was an annual incidence rate of two HP cases for every million members of the population. Of these, 83% of cases were organic, of these two-thirds were bacterial or fungal and one-third were related to animal protein exposures. The other 17% related to chemical exposure, particularly isocyanates.[33]

Much work has been done to describe a genetic explanation of host factors that predispose to development of HP in patients with antigen exposure. When compared with subjects who were either exposed to antigen with no reaction or not exposed at all, patients with antigen exposure and development of pigeon breeder's disease (a relatively common form of HP) were noted to have increased genetic variability in major histocompatibility complex and tumor necrosis factor-α haplotypes. This suggests a possible relationship between increased predisposition for inflammatory reaction and the development of HP.[34]

The pathophysiology of HP is a complex series of events connecting an antigenic stimulus to alveolar lymphocytosis and lung damage. Principally, patients with disposition for development of HP are exposed to inhaled antigen with resultant

Table 1
Comparing WRA to HP

	HP	"Sensitizer-induced" OA
Pathophysiology	Antigen sensitization followed by IgG-mediated type-4 hypersensitivity response and alveolar lymphocytosis resulting in alveolar and interstitial fibrosis	Antigen sensitization followed by IgE-mediated type-1 hypersensitivity response and eosinophilic airway infiltration consistent with other types of asthma
Clinical presentation	Dyspnea or cough after exposure to trigger substance	Dyspnea or cough with or without wheeze after exposure to trigger substance
Radiograph	Bilateral ground-glass opacities with centrilobular nodularity on chest tomogram	Generally unremarkable
Spirometry	Nonspecific Mixed obstruction early in the course with progression to restriction as fibrosis becomes more severe	Obstructive physiology with positive bronchodilator response
Treatment	Antigen avoidance with steroid bursts as necessary	Antigen avoidance with inhaled-corticosteroids and bronchodilator therapy, as in other types of asthma

sensitization. Re-exposure prompts antibody formation and alveolar CD8+ lymphocyte activation with subsequent lung damage related to alveolitis.[35] Patients with a history of tobacco inhalation have decreased rates of HP, suggestive of an immunomodulatory effect resulting in decreased alveolitis. Risk of developing summer-type HP, a prevalent subset of HP related to mold found in Japanese homes, was greater in housemates of known HP patients who did not smoke than in smokers exposed to the same risk.[36] This may relate to the known diminution of alveolar lymphocyte activity in cigarette smokers.[37] Changes related to lymphocytic alveolar damage are generally histopathologically identical to other autoimmune pneumonitides with the principal difference being the association of HP with evidence of antigen-related immune response. This association can be demonstrated either with serum antibodies to a known antigen or with *bronchoalveolar lavage* (BAL) fluid with lymphocytic infiltration (BAL with 30%–70% lymphocytes).[32]

Usually, pathologic analysis reveals inflammatory changes in the airways with alveolar lymphocytosis and interstitial monocytosis, as well as scattered nonnecrotizing granulomas. Radiographically, thoracic tomography demonstrates bilateral ground-glass opacities and/or centrilobular nodularity. If this cellular response persists and HP becomes chronic, pulmonary function testing may reveal classic restrictive physiology with an impaired diffusion of carbon monoxide, as in pigeon breeder's disease. However, airway inflammation may have the effect of increasing airway collapsibility resulting in obstructive physiology, as in farmer's lung.[38] As the changes associated with disease can affect alveoli, interstitia, and airways, there may be significant overlapping of obstructive and restrictive changes. Therefore, pulmonary function testing is nonspecific in the assessment of HP.

The clinical presentation of HP is variable depending on phase of disease, though there is significant overlap across the disease spectrum. Typically, acute HP presents with cough, dyspnea, and chest tightness within 12 hours of exposure to antigen and rapid resolution after exposure ceases. In patients who have transformed to subacute or chronic disease, presentation includes cough, dyspnea, and flu-like symptoms; however, these may persist even after immediate exposure has ended.[39] Physical examination will often reveal crackles but examination may remain normal in up to 20% of cases.[40]

Attempts at uniform diagnostic criteria have been made, but have largely been unsuccessful. In 2003, the Hypersensitivity Pneumonitis (HP) Study Group attempted to identify a clinical prediction rule for patients with HP. This study remains useful in determining the likelihood of this diagnosis in a patient with risk factors who describes a history of dyspnea and cough.[40] Six hundred and sixty-one patients with disease concerning for acute or subacute HP were evaluated. A committee of clinicians, radiologists, and pathologists determined the presence or absence of HP based on available evidence (BAL fluid, histopathology, radiographs, and clinical presentations). After comparing the group with HP to the group without HP, a comprehensive battery of objective findings was assessed. This resulted in a six-part predictive rule for increased likelihood of HP. The variables associated with increased likelihood were: (1) exposure to a known offending antigen, (2) presence of precipitating antibodies to the offending antigen, (3) recurrent symptoms, (4) inspiratory crackles on physical examination, (5) symptoms occurring 4 to 8 hours after exposure, and (6) weight loss. A prediction model was developed using combinations of variables to determine probability of having HP. Using this prediction rule, patients with intermediate likelihood for HP could be referred for further evaluation using radiologic and pathologic evidence to guide final diagnosis.

Therefore, as with much of medicine, the diagnosis of HP begins with a comprehensive medical history to include exposure to known antigenic triggers. Some common triggers include bird feathers, isocyanates (used in some commercial pesticides), rotten wood, metalworking fluids, hot tubs, and dairy barns.[32] Symptoms may resolve when the trigger is withdrawn though this is less reliable with advanced disease. Radiography and histology will be nonspecific but may include the typical changes described above.

A rational approach to the evaluation in a patient at risk includes taking a detailed history followed by pulmonary function testing and high-resolution CT evaluation of the lung parenchyma to evaluate for consistent changes or an alternative diagnosis. In patients with several of the indicators listed above and consistent radiographic changes, workup should include measurement of serum antibodies of interest and bronchoalveolar lavage to evaluate for lymphocyte prominence and microbiologic organisms (to include mycobacteria and fungi).

The outcomes of patients with HP are closely linked to the duration of exposure, the delay in diagnosis, and the ability of the patient to avoid further exposure. Although simply ceasing exposure to the offending antigen will result in improvement in many patients, those with advanced disease (fibrosis or obstructive changes) may not experience clinical remission after withdrawal. Treatment beyond antigenic avoidance is primarily limited to steroid therapy in bursts surrounding symptom development or chronically in patients with advanced disease. The usefulness of inhaled bronchodilators and alternative immunomodulators has yet to be defined in trials with adequate power to guide therapeutic planning.

CHURG-STRAUSS SYNDROME

Churg-Strauss syndrome (CSS) is a necrotizing, antineutrophil cytoplasmic antibody (ANCA)-associated small-vessel to medium-vessel vasculitis with a predilection for involvement of respiratory mucosa and a prominent eosinophilia.[41] The prevalence is estimated at 10.7 to 14 cases per million adults with an annual new incidence rate of 0.1 to 2.6 cases per million.[42]

CSS typically follows a triphasic progress with an initial prodromal phase consisting of rhinosinusitis and asthma followed by a peripheral eosinophilia with myocardial, gastrointestinal, and pulmonary involvement. The final phase is a progression to systemic vasculitis with development of dermatologic, neurologic, and renal involvement.[43]

Between 95% and 100% of patients with CSS will report symptoms of dyspnea, cough, and wheeze early in the course of their disease. Asthma symptoms in CSS are typically adult-onset and often refractory to traditional therapy with frequent need for systemic corticosteroid support. In the prodromal phase, patients may also note comorbid nasal polyps, frequent allergic rhinitis, and chronic sinusitis.[42] The development of progressively increasing peripheral eosinophilia and visceral involvement heralds the second phase of disease. Prominent features during this phase involve increased pulmonary infiltration, gastrointestinal upset, and myocardial involvement. Some investigators hypothesize that the use of steroids early in asthma may delay onset of vasculitic symptoms in CSS.

CSS remains predominantly a clinical diagnosis with radiologic, laboratory, and pathologic evidence supporting the clinical findings (**Box 3**). Diagnostic criteria, developed in 1990, include the presence of asthma, more than 10% peripheral blood eosinophils, mononeuropathy multiplex or polyneuropathy, nonfixed pulmonary infiltrates, paranasal sinus abnormality, and extravascular eosinophils on a biopsy including a blood vessel. The presence of four out of these six criteria yielded an 85% sensitivity and 99.7% specificity for CSS. The same group devised a classification tree which allowed for classification of CSS in patients with peripheral eosinophilia and either asthma or a documented non-asthma, non-drug reaction allergy. This system yielded a 95% sensitivity and 99.2% specificity.[44] Additionally, approximately 40% of patients with CSS demonstrate serologic evidence of elevated perinuclear-ANCAs against myeloperoxidase.[41] BAL often demonstrates a normal cell count but an increased prevalence of eosinophils, whereas lung biopsy may reveal eosinophilic pneumonia with or without granuloma formation.[42] Radiographic findings are variable but, most commonly, involve transient, bilateral, noncavitary infiltrates.

Before the use of corticosteroids, CSS had a mortality of approximately 50%.[42] In some modern series, remission was noted in as many as 91% of patients with CSS.[45] Therapeutic attempts to induce remission in patients with CSS have generally involved a combination of pulse-dose corticosteroids and alternative

---

Box 3
Diagnostic criteria for CSS

Four or more of these six criteria yields 85% sensitivity and 99.7% specificity for CSS

- Presence of asthma
- Greater than 10% peripheral blood eosinophils
- Mononeuropathy multiplex or polyneuropathy
- Nonfixed pulmonary infiltrates
- Paranasal sinus abnormality
- Extravascular eosinophils on a biopsy including a blood vessel

immunosuppressants with the goal of decreased chronic steroid burden. This can be accomplished with intravenous methylprednisolone coadministered with cyclophos-phamide or methotrexate in patients with markers of poor prognosis. In patients without markers of poor prognosis, induction of remission may be accomplished with oral prednisone alone. Maintenance of immunosuppression can be achieved with methotrexate, cyclosporine, or azathioprine.[42] A five-factor score has been devel-oped to predict mortality and guide therapy in patients with CSS, including (1) protein-uria greater than 1 g per day, (2) myocardial vasculitic involvement, (3) severe GI involvement (perforation, pancreatitis, bleeding), (4) heart disease, and (5) a short duration of the asthmatic phase of disease. These were all independently associated with worse outcomes.[45] These patients are at higher risk of mortality and should have alterations in therapy guided toward aggressive immunosuppression as tolerated.

CSS is a clinical diagnosis describing a syndrome of eosinophilic vasculitis that frequently presents in early stages with asthma and allergic symptoms. Given the poten-tial for increased mortality if diagnosis is delayed until the vasculitic phase, it is critical for all practitioners involved in the care of asthmatics to maintain awareness of the disease and pursue additional workup in patients fulfilling multiple diagnostic criteria for CSS.

ALLERGIC BRONCHOPULMONARY ASPERGILLOSIS

Allergic bronchopulmonary aspergillosis (ABPA) represents a multi-type airway hyper-sensitivity response to *Aspergillus* species. A mixed response consisting of allergic (type 1), immune complex (type 3), and cell-mediated (type 4) components results in episodic bronchial obstruction, peripheral eosinophilia, antigen-specific skin test positivity, presence of serum antibodies, elevated IgE concentrations, and central bronchiectasis with pulmonary infiltration on radiography.[46,47] Despite having a prev-alence of 1% to 2% among patients with asthma (2%–15% in cystic fibrosis), the diag-nostic latency is often as long as 10 years.[48] Given the potential therapeutic options if diagnosis occurs promptly, and the potential harm of delay, it is imperative that all physicians routinely treating chronic asthma recognize the significance of this patho-logic condition and the proper approach to treatment.

ABPA develops when genetically susceptible individuals are exposed to environ-mental *Aspergillus* species, which become trapped in viscous sputum with a resulting surge in cellular and cytokinetic inflammatory response. Mucociliary clearance is impaired, a Th-2 cytokine response occurs, and antigen-specific IgE is synthesized. Progressively, these events promote mast cell degranulation, eosinophilic proliferanation, and characteristic pathologic changes of asthma, including bronchial interstitial eosinophilia.[46]

Patients with ABPA will typically present with difficult-to-control asthma with classic symptoms of dyspnea, cough, chest tightness, and occasional wheeze. Although not particularly sensitive, the finding of brownish sputum in a chronic asthmatic raises the concern for ABPA. Asthmatic patients presenting with difficult-to-control symptoms, expectoration of mucus plugs, fever, or weight loss should be screened.[46] For a diag-nosis of ABPA, patients should have immediate cutaneous reactivity to *Aspergillus*, an elevated serum IgE concentration, and specific anti-*Aspergillus* immunoglobulins.[48] Some patients will also have radiographic bronchiectasis in the proximal airways, though this is not specific. Pleural thickening, transient infiltrates, consolidation, and atelectasis can be observed. Sputum cultures may be falsely negative and the pres-ence of *Aspergillus* in sputum may occur in patients without ABPA.

A nonlinear, five-stage system for grading the severity of ABPA, developed in the 1980s, describes the spectrum of disease ranging from acute symptoms through remission, exacerbation, corticosteroid-dependent asthma, and fibrotic disease.[49] On diagnosis, therapy is initiated with eradication of environmental molds, treatment of comorbid sinusitis and/or gastroesophageal reflux disease, and initiation of systemic corticosteroids. Corticosteroid dose adjustment is based on improvements in spirometry, IgE level, radiography, and clinical symptoms.[48] Once the prednisone dose is less than 10 mg per day, one may consider alternating to (or adding) inhaled corticosteroids.[46] Although itraconazole is the best studied antifungal for the management of ABPA, controversy exists whether its proper role is as a primary, steroid-sparing therapy or as an adjunct to steroids in severely ill patients.[47,48]

SUMMARY

The symptoms of asthma may represent a variety of underlying pathologic processes. In patients whose asthma history is vague or whose treatment response is suboptimal to conventional therapy, the extended differential diagnosis must be considered. This article has introduced some of the more common disease processes associated with the development of wheeze, cough, or shortness of breath. Increased awareness should result in increased efforts to identify alternative processes and address the actual underlying pathologic condition. Through these efforts, symptomatic relief may be achieved in a greater proportion of patients with asthma or its mimickers.

REFERENCES

1. Han JK. Subclassification of chronic rhinosinusitis. Laryngoscope 2013; 123(Suppl 2):S15–27.
2. Moebus RG, Han JK. Immunomodulatory treatments for aspirin exacerbated respiratory disease. Am J Rhinol Allergy 2012;26(2):134–40.
3. Higashi N, Taniguchi M, Mita H, et al. Clinical features of asthmatic patients with increased urinary leukotriene E4 excretion (hyperleukotrienuria): involvement of chronic hyperplastic rhinosinusitis with nasal polyposis. J Allergy Clin Immunol 2004;113(2):277–83.
4. Szczeklik A, Nizankowska E, Duplaga M. Natural history of aspirin-induced asthma. AIANE Investigators. European network on aspirin-induced asthma. Eur Respir J 2000;16(3):432–6.
5. Berges-Gimeno MP, Simon RA, Stevenson DD. The natural history and clinical characteristics of aspirin-exacerbated respiratory disease. Ann Allergy Asthma Immunol 2002;89(5):474–8.
6. Lee RU, Stevenson DD. Aspirin-exacerbated respiratory disease: evaluation and management. Allergy Asthma Immunol Res 2011;3(1):3–10.
7. Kowalski ML, Grzelewska-Rzymowska I, Szmidt M, et al. Clinical efficacy of aspirin in "desensitised" aspirin-sensitive asthmatics. Eur J Respir Dis 1986; 69(4):219–25.
8. Berges-Gimeno MP, Simon RA, Stevenson DD. Long-term treatment with aspirin desensitization in asthmatic patients with aspirin-exacerbated respiratory disease. J Allergy Clin Immunol 2003;111(1):180–6.
9. McMains KC, Kountakis SE. Medical and surgical considerations in patients with Samter's triad. Am J Rhinol 2006;20(6):573–6.
10. White A, Ludington E, Mehra P, et al. Effect of leukotriene modifier drugs on the safety of oral aspirin challenges. Ann Allergy Asthma Immunol 2006;97(5): 688–93.
11. Mantor PC, Tuggle DW, Tunell WP. An appropriate negative bronchoscopy rate in suspected foreign body aspiration. Am J Surg 1989;158(6):622–4.

12. Midulla F, Guidi R, Barbato A, et al. Foreign body aspiration in children. Pediatr Int 2005;47(6):663–8.
13. Karakoc F, Cakir E, Ersu R, et al. Late diagnosis of foreign body aspiration in children with chronic respiratory symptoms. Int J Pediatr Otorhinolaryngol 2007;71(2):241–6.
14. Dicpinigaitis PV. Chronic cough due to asthma: ACCP evidence-based clinical practice guidelines. Chest 2006;129:75S–9S.
15. Niimi A, Matsumoto H, Minakuchi M, et al. Airway remodeling in cough variant asthma. Lancet 2000;356:564–5.
16. Abouzgheib W, Pratter MR, Bartter T. Cough and asthma. Curr Opin Pulm Med 2007;13:44–8.
17. Dicpinigaitis PV, Dobkin JB, Reichel J. Antitussive effect of the leukotriene receptor antagonist zafirlukast in subjects with cough-variant asthma. J Asthma 2002; 39(4):291–7.
18. Desai D, Brightling C. Cough due to asthma. Cough-variant asthma and non-asthmatic eosinophilic bronchitis. Otolaryngol Clin North Am 2010;43: 123–30.
19. Fujimura M, Nishizawa Y, Nishitsuji M, et al. Predictors for typical asthma onset from cough variant asthma. J Asthma 2005;42:107–11.
20. De Diego A, Martinez E, Perpina M, et al. Airway inflammation and cough sensitivity in cough-variant asthma. Allergy 2005;60:1407–11.
21. Brightling CE, Ward R, Goh KL, et al. Eosinophilic bronchitis is an important cause of chronic cough. Am J Respir Crit Care Med 1999;160:406–10.
22. Brightling CE. Chronic cough due to nonasthmatic eosinophilic bronchitis: ACCP evidence-based clinical practice. Chest 2006;129:116S–21S.
23. Brightling CE, Ward R, Wardlaw AJ, et al. Airway inflammation, airway responsiveness and cough before and after inhaled budesonide in patients with eosinophilic bronchitis. Eur Respir J 2000;15:682–6.
24. Malo J, Vandenplas O. Definitions and classification of work-related asthma. Immunol Allergy Clin North Am 2011;31:645–62.
25. Tarlo SM, Balmes J, Balkissoon R, et al. Diagnosis and management of work-related asthma: American College of Chest Physicians Consensus Statement. Chest 2008;134:1S–41S.
26. Bakerly ND, Moore VC, Vellore AD, et al. Fifteen-year trends in occupational asthma: data from the shield surveillance scheme. Occup Med (Lond) 2008; 58:169–74.
27. Kenyon NJ, Morrissey BM, Schivo MAS, et al. Occupational asthma. Clin Rev Allergy Immunol 2012;43:3–13.
28. Baur X, Aasen TB, Burge PS, et al. The management of work-related asthma guidelines: a broader perspective. Eur Respir Rev 2012;21:124–39.
29. Anees W, Gannon PF, Huggins V, et al. Effect of peak expiratory flow data quantity on diagnostic sensitivity and specificity in occupational asthma. Eur Respir J 2004;23:730–4.
30. Beach J, et al. Diagnosis and management of work-related asthma: summary. AHRQ evidence report summaries. Rockville (MD): Agency for Healthcare Research and Quality (US); 2005. p. 129, 1998-2005. Available at: http://www.ncbi.nlm.nih.gov/books/NBK11926/.
31. Lemiere C, Pizzichini MM, Balkissoon R, et al. Diagnosing occupational asthma: use of induced sputum. Eur Respir J 1999;13:482–8.
32. Lacasse Y, Girard M, Cormier Y. Recent advances in hypersensitivity pneumonitis. Chest 2012;142(1):208–17.

33. McDonald JC, Chen Y, Zekveld C, et al. Incidence by occupation and industry of acute work related respiratory disease in the United Kingdom. 1992–2001. Occup Environ Med 2005;62:836–42.

34. Camarena A, Juárez A, Mejía M, et al. Major histocompatibility complex and tumor necrosis factor-α polymorphisms in Pigeon Breeder's Disease. Am J Respir Crit Care Med 2001;163:1528–33.

35. Prince JE, Kheradmand F, Corry DB. Chapter 16: immunologic lung disease. J Allergy Clin Immunol 2003;111:S613–23.

36. Arima K, Ando M, Ito K, et al. Effect of cigarette smoking on prevalence of summer-type hypersensitivity pneumonitis caused by Trichosporon cutaneum. Arch Environ Health 1992;47(4):274–8.

37. Sopori M. Effects of cigarette smoke on the immune system. Nat Rev Immunol 2002;2(5):372–7.

38. Lalancette M, Carrier G, Laviolette M, et al. Farmer's lung. Long-term outcome and lack of predictive value of bronchoalveolar lavage fibrosing factors. Am Rev Respir Dis 1993;148(1):216–21.

39. Hanak V, Golbin JM, Ryu JH. Causes and presenting features in 85 consecutive patients with hypersensitivity pneumonitis. Mayo Clin Proc 2007;82(7):812–6.

40. Lacasse Y, Selman M, Costabel U, et al. Clinical diagnosis of hypersensitivity pneumonitis. Am J Respir Crit Care Med 2003;168(8):952–8.

41. Abril A. Churg-Strauss syndrome: an update. Curr Rheumatol Rep 2011;13(6):488–95.

42. Baldini C, Talarico R, Della Rossa A, et al. Clinical manifestations and treatment of Churg-Strauss syndrome. Rheum Dis Clin North Am 2010;36(3):527–43.

43. Lanham JG. Systemic vasculitis with asthma and eosinophilia: a clinical approach to the Churg–Strauss syndrome. Medicine 1984;63:65–81.

44. Masi AT, Hunder GG, Lie JT, et al. The American College of Rheumatology 1990 criteria for the classification of Churg-Strauss syndrome (allergic granulomatosis and angiitis). Arthritis Rheum 1990;33(8):1094–100.

45. Guillevin L, Cohen P, Gayraud M, et al. Churg-Strauss syndrome. Clinical study and long-term follow-up of 96 patients. Medicine 1999;78(1):26–37.

46. Agarwal R. Allergic bronchopulmonary aspergillosis. Chest 2009;135:805–26.

47. Walsh TJ, Anaissie EJ, Denning DW, et al. Treatment of aspergillosis: clinical practice guidelines of the Infectious Diseases Society of America. Clin Infect Dis 2008;46(3):327–60.

48. Greenberger PA. Allergic bronchopulmonary aspergillosis. J Allergy Clin Immunol 2002;110:685–92.

49. Patterson R, Greenberger PA, Radin RC, et al. Allergic bronchopulmonary aspergillosis: staging as an aid to management. Ann Intern Med 1982;96:286–91.

Index

Note: Page numbers of article titles are in **boldface** type.

Moving?

Make sure your subscription moves with you!

To notify us of your new address, find your **Clinics Account Number** (located on your mailing label above your name), and contact customer service at:

Email: journalscustomerservice-usa@elsevier.com

800-654-2452 (subscribers in the U.S. & Canada)
314-447-8871 (subscribers outside of the U.S. & Canada)

Fax number: 314-447-8029

Elsevier Health Sciences Division
Subscription Customer Service
3251 Riverport Lane
Maryland Heights, MO 63043

ELSEVIER

Printed and bound by CPI Group (UK) Ltd, Croydon, CR0 4YY

16/10/2024

01774857-0001